A GUIDE TO LEGA
DESTINATIONS AC

GREEN SCENES

LAUREN YOSHIKO

GREEN

GREEN

GREEN

GREEN

SCENES

LAUREN YOSHIKO

Hardie Grant

EXPLORE

WEST COAST

THE SOUTH-WEST

THE MID-WEST

EAST COAST

There was a time not so long ago that writing an article about marijuana meant risking your entire career—if not a lot more. For me, that time was early 2014, when I was writing weed columns for a Portland, Oregon alt-weekly under a pen name.

Oregonians ended up voting to legalize cannabis for adults twenty-one and older later that year, but until that point, it felt like a serious gamble to risk a comfortable desk job, the respect of bigger media outlets, and the approval of certain friends and family members to see my name associated with articles that revealed my degree of experience with the plant. I ended up dropping the pseudonym a year later, embracing the new editorial beat as the legalization wave continued down the West Coast. I eventually found additional work in the industry, running dispensaries and working at cannabis farms to pay the bills.

Contemporary cannabis culture continued to blossom, as did my writing career. Each newly legalized state brought in new readers and story angles. "Cannabis" became the new-world term for the plant, and I found myself moderating cannabis panels from Portland to Montreal, observing the way its stigma ebbed and flowed across the continent as those with cannabis-related charges struggled to get justice. Over the course of my hundreds of interviews with growers, edible chefs, wellness practitioners, artists, and entrepreneurs, I noticed that the deeper the pockets and cleaner the criminal record, the much higher likelihood of accessing and succeeding in this new world of legal weed.

I also noticed that, across the board, most of the people entering this industry with the desire to share the good this plant can do—both when consumed and as a potential model for ethical business practices—did so with little more than their bootstraps. I learned how much every purchase counts, how we, as weed lovers, played a vital role in deciding which businesses had a fighting chance against venture capital-funded corporations set on

INTROD

turning legal weed into another Big Tobacco. So I've dedicated much of the past ten years to highlighting the folks going the extra mile to build an industry of thriving, small, diverse businesses that put the well-being of people and planet before profits.

The following pages are home to some of the most interesting dispensaries, hemp-friendly spaces, and cannabis-centric experiences and lodging across fifteen states. Almost all are locally owned, and every single one is operated by people who care about the healing properties of the plant, the positive disruptive potential of the industry, and the well-being of their employees. Every destination included in these pages is fully legal, meaning they are all licensed shops in good standing with state regulations or experiences operating within the unique laws of their state. Additionally, each of these businesses is open for adults over the age of twenty-one—no medical card or patient registration required.

You will find that some legal states are not featured extensively here, and that's because scenes take time to develop. The amount of red tape one needs to get through—from submitting an application to navigating licensing processes; getting spots approved, inspected, and opened; and establishing a community—can easily take multiple years after voters legalize. For now, the states included here are home to the most dynamic legal cannabis scenes in the country.

Depending on where your adventures take you, there may be a dozen other shops closer than the ones mentioned here. Regardless of who you choose to patronize, I hope this book empowers you to spend your dollars on the farms and brands you want to see succeed within cannabis scenes and beyond.

LAUREN YOSHIKO

UCTION

WEED

A glossary of cannabis vocabulary, product types, industry terms, common slang, and colloquial nicknames that might prove useful as you navigate this newly legal realm.

CANNABINOID

The influential compounds that contribute to cannabis's effect on the body and mind. THC (tetrahydrocannabinol) is a cannabinoid, as is CBD (cannabidiol). We only understand a fraction of the 113 distinct cannabinoids identified so far, but we do know they interact with our bodies in a range of profound ways.

CANNABIS

Marijuana, weed, pot, grass, bud, flower, herb—all words for the same plant. "Cannabis" has become the most commonly used word within the industry, but you can call it whatever you want!

CANNA-BUTTER

The classic method of slow-cooking weed in butter in order to pull the cannabinoids and other plant compounds from the leaves. Those fatty compounds bind with the fats of the butter, so once you remove the excess plant material, the remaining butter is ready to be used in a batch of very special brownies.

CONCENTRATE

Extract, oil, hash—all of these terms refer to the sticky, potent concentration of resin one can draw off of the cannabis plant leaves and consume on its own. Think of it a bit like what maple syrup is to a maple tree. There are many types of concentrates that all differ in texture, potency, and flavor, but their main differences come down to two things: the method of processing and the source material (e.g., whole buds versus leaf bits and stems). All are typically consumed via dab or vape, but various types can be incorporated into edibles and "infused pre-rolls." Here are some popular types of concentrates you may come across:

BHO, or butane hash oil: This concentrate is made using pressurized chemical solvents, like butane, to strip cannabis's essential oils from the plant matter within a closed-loop system. It sounds gnarly, but dabbers love this stuff because of the flavor.

CO_2 OIL: This is a form of concentrate that's extracted from the plant by running it through a machine that uses pressure and carbon dioxide to separate and isolate cannabinoids and other essential compounds. Carbon dioxide is a common solvent used for pharmaceutical extraction and processes like decaffeinating coffee.

RESIN: This is a concentrate made with fresh, whole flower (as opposed to the leftover leaf bits trimmed off of the plant—called "trim"—commonly used for concentrates) via CO2 extraction or using a solvent like butane. You might hear the term "live resin," which refers to resin made from flash-frozen buds, which helps retain more flavor.

ROSIN: If we think of hash as the results of hand-squeezing an orange, rosin is what you get with a precise, mechanized juice press. Hash is made from gathering the outer compounds that cling to leaves and buds, but the combination of heat and pressure further breaks down the compounds that are further sieved one more time, resulting in this more pure, potent, and botanically rich concentrate.

RSO: Rick Simpson Oil (RSO) is named after the Canadian hospital engineer who successfully treated his skin cancer using a homemade cannabis concoction made by soaking cannabis in pure alcohol. Also known as Phoenix Tears, RSO can be applied directly to the skin or eaten like an edible.

DAB

Not to be confused with the dance move, a dab is both a single hit of concentrate and the verb associated with consuming it. Because of its potency, only a tiny "dab" of concentrate suffices, which is heated in a glass pipe or vape pen—called a "dab rig"—to a hot enough temperature for the concentrate to transform into inhalable vapor.

DISPENSARY

A state-licensed cannabis retail store or provisioning center. Learn how to shop at one on pages xii-xiii.

WORDS

EDIBLES

Food, candy, and beverages that contain cannabis.

ENDOCANNABINOID SYSTEM (ECS)

A complex network of chemical signals and cellular receptors found throughout our brains and bodies. The ECS plays a role in many processes that affect our daily lives, including our mood, circadian rhythms, intestinal strength, metabolism, pain tolerance, and much more. This system is what interacts with cannabinoids in cannabis to induce a high when we consume it.

FLOWER

Also known as buds or "nugs," this describes the part of the cannabis plant that is dried, cured, and trimmed to smokable perfection.

HEMP

Because of the separation of hemp and cannabis laws, we treat them as two different plants. In reality, though, the cannabis plant comes in an incredibly wide range of potencies, and the ones with very little THC—less than 0.3% by federal definition—are considered hemp plants.

INDICA

This, as well as sativa, is a popular way to categorize cannabis into two types: relaxing, mellowing strains referred to as "indica," and uplifting, stimulating strains known as "sativa." Cannabis strains can't really be accurately separated into such a simple dichotomy, as a strain that puts me to sleep might hit one of you as a nice day high, and vice versa.

KIEF

This is the glittery, light green, sticky powder that collects on your fingertips when you handle properly cured flower or in the recesses of the grinder when buds are ground up.

SOCIAL EQUITY

Social equity is fair, impartial justice for all people, and in the cannabis industry, this term encompasses both accounting for systemic inequalities to ensure equal access to opportunities and the righting of wrongs committed over the course of racially biased cannabis prohibition. Because the elements and programs dedicated to these efforts often go by "social equity," industry workers licensed through these programs often go by the title "equity operators."

STRAIN

Think of a cannabis strain (aka cultivar) as a plant varietal, like the way champagne is a type of wine. You could say roma, red beefsteak, heirloom, and cherry are all different tomato "strains." Also, similarly to the way some batches of roma will taste sweeter or more robust than others, depending on the seed genetics and the methods of the farmers, two batches of the same strain won't necessarily feel identical.

A note regarding strain names: The cannabis industry has been cross-breeding cannabis plants more fervently than corn, apples, and soybeans combined over the past fifty years—and none of that has been tracked or collated in any shared database. One man's Blue Dream might feel like another's Sundae Driver. I recommend following farms you like more than strains you like, as each farm's methods will likely deliver consistently satisfying effects across their varieties.

SUBLINGUALS

These are edibles that absorb through the tissue under the tongue like lozenges or mouth sprays. These typically have a faster onset of effects than eating and metabolizing an edible brownie.

TERPENE

Terpenes are naturally occurring compounds that prominently contribute to the aroma and flavor of cannabis. They have some degree of effect on how different strains affect different people as well.

TINCTURES

A liquid concentrate procured through steam alcohol extraction, which pulls out the plant's beneficial cannabinoids and is concentrated down to a very medicinally potent liquid that can be consumed or applied topically to the skin.

TRIM

The bits of leaf cut away from the plant during post-harvest pruning before it hits shelves. Trim is typically sold to a processor, which then extracts the good stuff for use in edibles, vape pens, and other concentrate products.

VAPE

A vape, or vaporizer, heats cannabis flower or concentrate until it releases its active components into a vapor that can be inhaled. Since the plant isn't combusted with fire, your lungs aren't getting hit with carcinogens like they do when you light up a joint or pipe. Different styles of vapes can include vape pens with disposable cartridges, disposable vape pens, handheld refillable vapes, and standalone vaporizers like the renowned Volcano.

HOW TO SHOP AT A

WHAT TO BRING

Government-issued identification, like a driver's license or passport, for example. A Costco card will not get you into a dispensary.

Cash. The whole federally illegal thing continues to halt federally insured banks or credit providers from paying for legal cannabis transactions. Most dispensaries will have an ATM on site, which typically have $1–5 withdrawal fees. Just bring cash.

WHEN YOU ARRIVE

Depending on the state and business, there may be security guards out front, and depending on the state, they could be armed. This is a "normal" security precaution at US dispensaries, and in some cities, it's required. As soon as you're inside, prepare to show your ID again. This isn't like going to a bar and hanging toward the back, hoping no one cards you. You will get carded whether you look under twenty-one or over eighty.

MEET YOUR BUDTENDER

When medical dispensaries were getting established, the employees started going by the name "budtender," and this riff on "bartender" has stuck ever since. Some feel the term has a slightly negative connotation, tying it to stereotypes of dispensary employees being less professional stoners. However, as someone who worked at a dispensary in the past and witnessed the powerful experience of connecting a customer with the product that improves their quality of life, I believe that people who work at dispensaries deserve their own unique term. I use the title budtender with utmost reverence and pride.

FIRST TIME? TELL THEM!

Ask questions! Tell them why you're there, be it your first time visit, a specific pain issue or concern, or just out of curiosity, and they'll leave you alone or start navigating you to the right section of the store. You don't need to educate yourself in cannabis science in order to shop for weed, but coming in with a clear idea of what you're looking for will make a huge difference.

SHOPPING TIME

While budtenders are not licensed medical professionals, they do know their products. They've sampled at least half of the products in the store, and they listen to testimonials all day, every day. At this point in cannabis research, they are as well equipped to guide you toward products that are most likely to deliver the desired effects as anyone else. Every cannabis strain and product will affect an individual differently due to their unique body chemistry, so you can't necessarily take any recommendation as a sure thing.

One thing you can do is trust your nose. Much of the effects of cannabis are determined by terpenes, the fragrant compounds that appear all over nature and contribute to aroma and effects. If a strain smells good to you, that's a good sign. If it doesn't smell good to you, or even makes you want to sneeze, that could be your body saying, "Next!" So when shopping in dispensaries that allow one to do so, take advantage and whiff away.

A note regarding prices: Cannabis taxes are significant. There are state, city, and often local taxes required on every transaction. Some stores factor them into the menu prices, and some will add them at the register, so brace yourself. If you want to experience a quality product that is crafted with care, it's good to acknowledge that those experiences may not exist on the budget shelf.

NO LIGHTING UP IN STORE

Unless the shop has a designated smoking lounge, you are not allowed to consume anything in store—before or after purchasing. Any samples at a legal shop will be "uninfused," as in virgin gummies that don't contain cannabis. You'll need to leave the store and find a private space out of public view to consume your newly acquired goodies.

BE KIND — WE'RE ALL STILL FIGURING THIS OUT

I know showing your ID every time is annoying, but them's the rules. Patience is a virtue at dispensaries. State-mandated processes, unintuitive software, and clunky packaging requirements can make a simple transaction take a few minutes longer than normal—no matter how fast or experienced the dispensary employee may be. Plus, any extra grams of patience you can find may pay off in the form of a discount at checkout.

DISPENSARY

HOW TO SHOP AT A DISPENSARY

RNIA   OREGON   WASHINGTON   MO

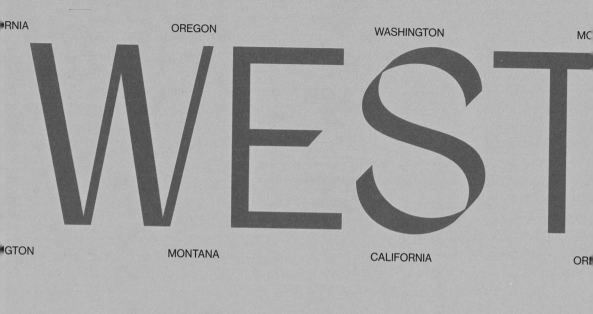

GTON   MONTANA   CALIFORNIA   OR

RNIA   OREGON   WASHINGTON   MOI

GTON   MONTANA   CALIFORNIA   ORE

CALIFORNIA

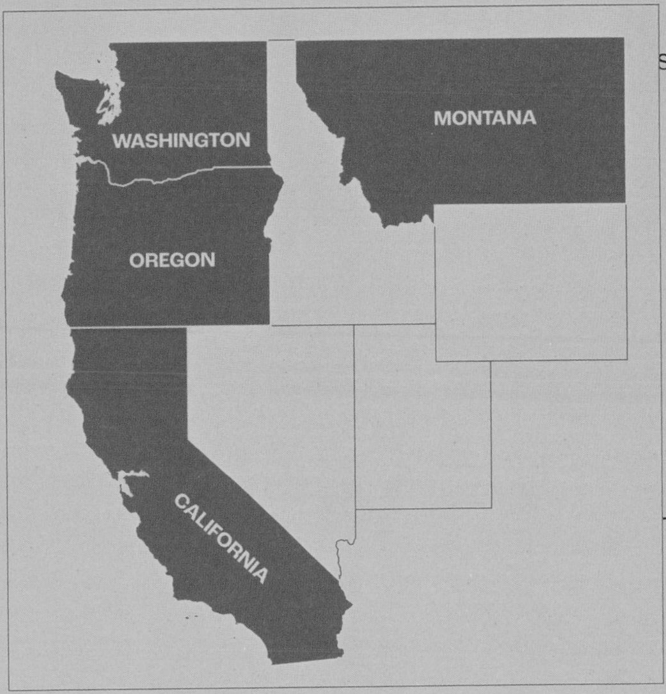

SHIN

WASHINGTON

LIFOR

CALIFORNIA OREGON WASHIN

OAST

WASHINGTON MONTANA CALIFO

Even if you've never been to the US West Coast, you've likely associated cannabis with California at some point. Maybe it was when learning about 1960s counterculture and the Summer of Love, or perhaps while exploring the origins of skateboard and surfer culture. I found my affinity for the plant while getting my undergraduate degree in literature at the University of California at Santa Cruz, a campus where cannabis was the unofficial mascot, legal tender, and popular icebreaker of most social circles. Its creative embrace nurtured my writing voice as I scribbled whimsies and observations underneath dense boughs of Redwood trees between lectures.

Many weed-related roads lead back to the Emerald Triangle—the slightly triangular outline of Humboldt, Trinity, and Mendocino Counties in Northern California, where vast spreads of serene, uninhabited land drew in green-thumbed black sheep and wayward homesteaders from all over in the 1960s. Since then it has grown into the country's most robust cannabis-producing region, and those still growing on the hallowed grounds under the sun follow in the footsteps of the foremothers and fathers of today's cannabis culture. From the Emerald Triangle and San Francisco's hippie havens to Hollywood magic and wildly creative cannabis brands, the Golden State offers its own world of immersive weed experiences.

EUREKA   SAN FRANCISCO BAY AREA   LOS ANGELES   PALM SPRINGS

CALIFO

LEGALIZED

Medical in 1996, Recreational in 2016

POSSESSION

Adults over the age of twenty-one can possess: one ounce of cannabis flower and up to eight grams of cannabis concentrate-infused products like edible gummies or vape cartridges.

HOME GROWS

You can buy cannabis seeds (no legal limit) and grow up to six cannabis plants at home.

DELIVERY

Yes, but only to private residences (no hotels).

CONSUMPTION

Smoking is allowed on private property and in licensed consumption lounges.

CITIES

Eureka (Humboldt County)
San Francisco Bay Area
Los Angeles
Palm Springs
San Diego

SAN DIEGO   EUREKA   SAN FRANCISCO BAY AREA   LOS ANGELES

ORNIA

MOON MADE FARMS

A BELOVED WOMEN-OWNED, SUNGROWN, REGENERATIVE CULTIVATOR BASED IN THE EMERALD TRIANGLE.

Tina Gordon, founder and head cultivator of Moon Made Farms, is a sincere steward of the land and someone I've looked up to for years. When she started growing cannabis on a forty-acre parcel in Humboldt County, she planted the seeds among oak trees, flowers, and native herbs so they could soak up real sunlight and help maintain healthy soil between harvests. Today, the plants are watered with captured rainwater, and each crop's seeds are often planted under a springtime new moon—an ancient tradition that inspires the farm's name and is backed by moisture retention science.

The farm is Sun+Earth Certified, a distinction given to cannabis farms that are not only organic and chemical-free but take regular steps to maintain soil health, enhance the habitat for beneficial flora and fauna, treat employees fairly, and maintain a good relationship with the surrounding, non-cannabis community. In all of these ways, Gordon embodies a creative approach that factors in ancestral horticultural practices and modern science, always thinking of the well-being of the nature around her and the trends in millennial smoking circles.

At a time when indoor-grown flower is favored by dispensary buyers and under-informed consumers, Moon Made Farms is changing the narrative, demonstrating the satisfying qualities of sungrown flower that doesn't always look as crystallized and aesthetically perfect as indoor varieties. You can find Gordon's flower at dispensaries across the state and inside many pre-roll products and edible brands, like Drew Martin and Cosmic View, respectively. If you can't find her bud at your local dispensary, do your community a favor and suggest that the shop look into stocking it.

"The craft market is not represented in retail right now, but that's what people truly want and need," Gordon said. "It's the same reason people go to the farmers' market or a healthy grocer—the desire to nourish our bodies with real, nutrient-rich food."

moonmadefarms.com

Learn more about Sun + Earth Certification at sunandearth.org.

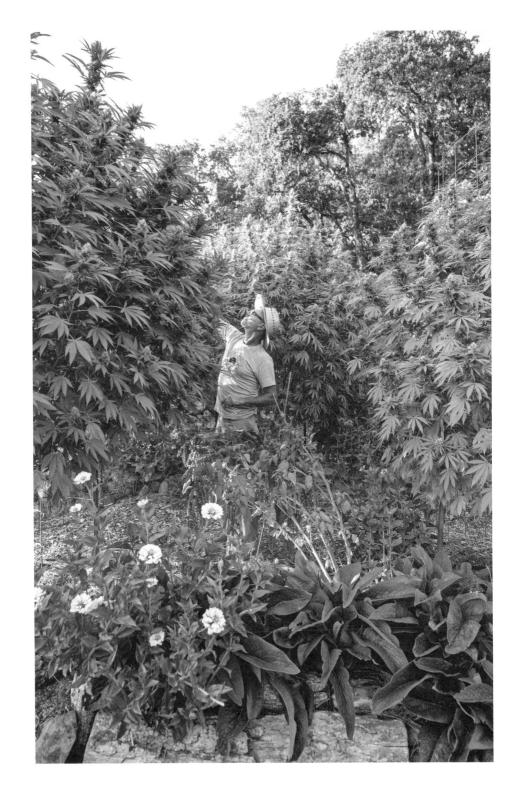

PAPA & BARKLEY SOCIAL

AN UPSCALE DISPENSARY AND CONSUMPTION LOUNGE AND SPA IN NORTHERN CALIFORNIA.

When cannabis was first legalized in California, the topicals from Papa & Barkley quickly became known throughout the state and beyond for their potency. In fact, it's the first California topical this little Oregonian tried, much to her satisfaction.

Named after founder Adam Grossman's father and his beloved pup, Papa & Barkley started with Grossman's desire to relieve his father's debilitating back pain. He got his hands on some quality cannabis, borrowed a slow cooker, and got to formulating the first version of their signature infused salve, Releaf Balm. The company has grown leaps and bounds since then while maintaining high standards for the cannabis that goes into their products.

They source sungrown hemp from carefully reviewed farms, with a focus on sustainable, regenerative farming practices that do not use pesticides or harmful chemicals. The flagship dispensary and lounge in Eureka offers customers an opportunity to experience their products on-site—an incredibly rare luxury in the maze of strict licensing rules. You can BYOC or shop Papa & Barkley body products and flower from four local, sungrown, women-run farms before heading to the outdoor consumption lounge to grab a spot by the fire pit. All that's missing are some barbecues—I'm already half inclined to host my next family reunion on-site.

I also recommend popping into the spa (yes, spa) for a chair massage. Call ahead to lean all the way in for a forty-five-minute couples massage that includes Papa & Barkley's rich THC-infused body oil. If you've got time, opt for The Entourage Effect: a ninety-minute, full-body massage complemented with a therapeutic terpene profile that is available for guests to inhale, ingest, and absorb throughout the massage.

Open Daily

4325 Broadway
Eureka, CA 95503

papaandbarkleysocial.com

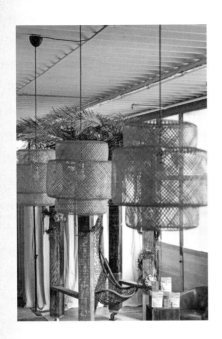

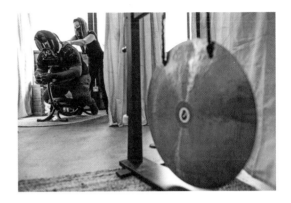

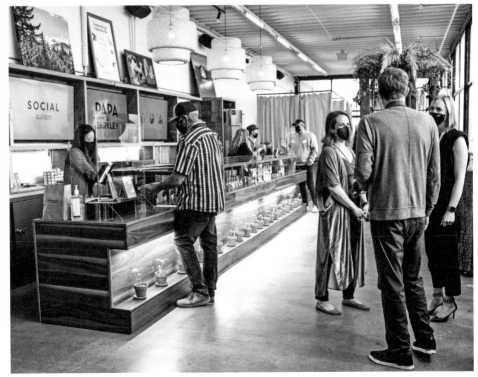

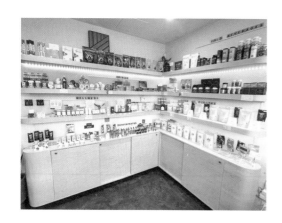

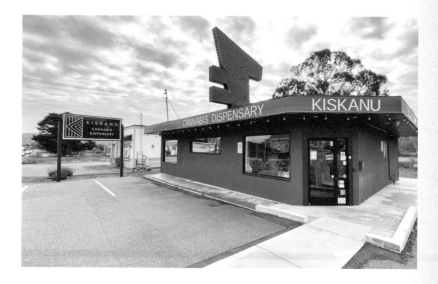

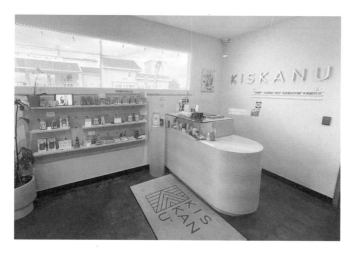

KISKANU

A FAMILY-RUN, VERTICALLY INTEGRATED BOUTIQUE DISPENSARY MAKING ITS OWN THC AND CBD TOPICALS.

Do you know what's more impressive than an independent dispensary selling house-grown flower? An independent dispensary that puts said house-grown flower into their own THC skincare *and* sexual wellness products (don't knock infused lube until you've tried it). Founders Gretchen and Jason Miller are lifelong cannabis cultivators who grew under California's medical marijuana program until 2018, when they started making cannabis-infused health and sexual wellness products for the legal market. During the buildout at their manufacturing site on Highway 101, they launched hemp CBD products, and in 2020, they made room for a cozy retail store in the front. They continue to grow THC flower in the sun on their Humboldt farm today—the Millers are about as legit as it gets.

Their topical lines feature face oil, intimacy oil, suppositories (reported by many to provide potent relief from menstrual and pelvic symptoms), and muscle rubs—all in THC and hemp CBD varieties. Most significantly, they're a family-owned brand supporting fellow NorCal businesses whenever possible. Alongside their Kiskanu flower, they carry Talking Trees Farms and Sunrise Mountain Farms—both longtime cultivators of sungrown and indoor flower—and edible companies like Space Gems, a local favorite for amazing vegan gummies made with solventless hash.

Open Daily

**2200 Fourth Street
Eureka, CA 95501**

kiskanudispensary.com

THE MADRONES INN AND THE BOHEMIAN CHEMIST

A RUSTIC CONSUMPTION-FRIENDLY INN WITH AN ON-SITE RESTAURANT AND DISPENSARY IN WINE COUNTRY.

Nestled in Anderson Valley, three hours south of Eureka, lies a one-of-a-kind oasis for cannabis lovers in the style of a Tuscan vineyard retreat. The Madrones Inn is a sprawling villa that includes three wine tasting rooms, luxurious guest accommodations, and a first-class restaurant with woodfired fare, while The Bohemian Chemist is a beautiful dispensary with decor and vibes straight out of the roaring 1920s. I'm a sucker for any kind of period-specific setting, and this Prohibition-esque apothecary delivers with vintage bottles, decanters, and art deco finds lining the walls of the warmly lit interior.

The dreamy property is flush with gardens, romantic gazebos, and twinkling lights strung among the redwoods and olive trees overhead. There is a designated consumption lounge on the property, and for those who opt to stay overnight, each suite features a private patio or deck where they can light up.

On top of this stunning boutique hotel, resort experience, and dispensary, co-owners Jim Roberts and Brian Adkinson also operate the house cannabis brand Sugarhill Farm. Their carefully sungrown flower is sold by the gram and in pre-rolls and vape cartridges at The Bohemian Chemist. It doesn't get more farm-to-table than that. Depending on the season, this eclectic compound also offers special cannabis-oriented weekend adventures, from infused dinners to farm tours and an annual craft cannabis auction.

Open Daily

**9000 Highway 128
Philo, CA 95466**

themadrones.com

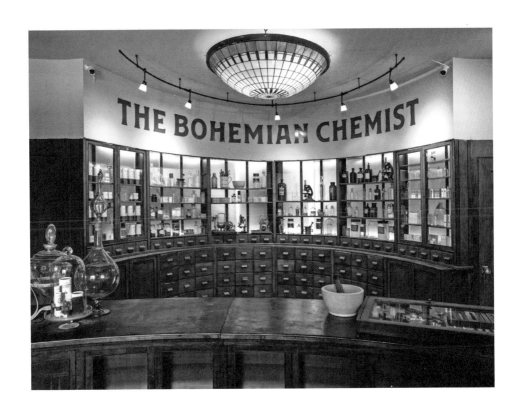

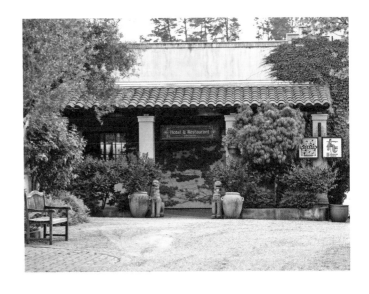

EMERALD FARM TOURS

NEXT-LEVEL CANNABIS TOURS SHOWING OFF THE BEST IN DOWNTOWN DISPENSARIES, RURAL FARMS, AND SPRAWLING WINE COUNTRY.

Emerald Farm Tours' famous Wine, Wilderness & Weed tour is more than a farm excursion. This eight-hour voyage takes guests to Mendocino County—also known as one third of the Emerald Triangle—where they get to walk among plants at a licensed cannabis farm and sample the region's produce straight from the people who grow it. Each tour is caringly led by Emerald Farm Tours co-founder Victor Pinho, who gives guests the lowdown on local cannabis culture as the bus ferries everyone over the Golden Gate Bridge, down picturesque Highway 101, and through vast expanses of Anderson Valley's vineyards.

There, guests can enjoy a full wine tasting and catered picnic before stopping at a family-run farm to wander among the plants, take photos, ask the growers questions, and learn about how cannabis goes from a living plant to a glittering, dried bud in a jar.

"Some people have emotional, almost spiritual experiences," Pinho said. "Standing in the shade of a towering cannabis plant for the first time and connecting it with the buds in their jar—I don't think they expect to be in the middle of nature instead of some warehouse. They're in the middle of a valley, the sun is shining, and the smell of cannabis hangs heavy in the air."

On the way back, the tour stops at The Bohemian Chemist dispensary, where guests can purchase cannabis grown in the valley they just strolled through. This Wine, Wilderness & Weed Tour is available every weekend in the summers until just past Labor Day, a time when sungrown cannabis plants are in full bloom ahead of harvest time in the fall. During the off-season, Pinho hosts simpler walking tours to two or three San Francisco dispensaries that, if guests choose, can include a cannabis-tasting experience at one of the city's consumption lounges.

Tours available daily

emeraldfarmtours.com

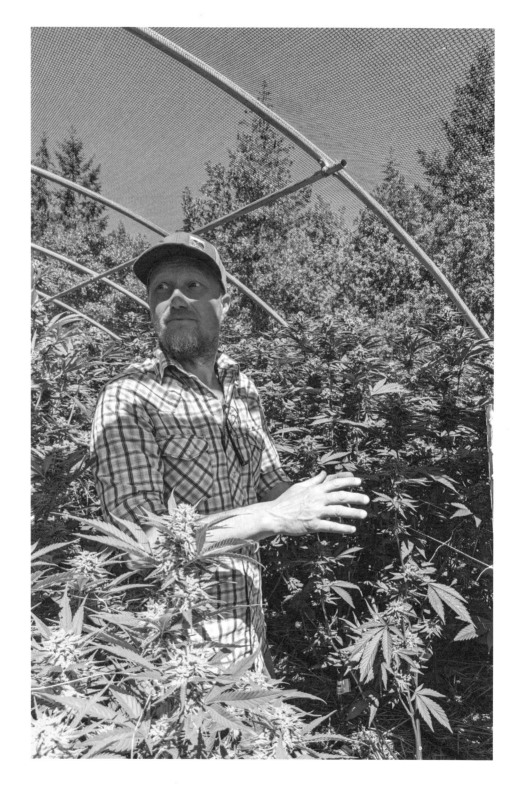

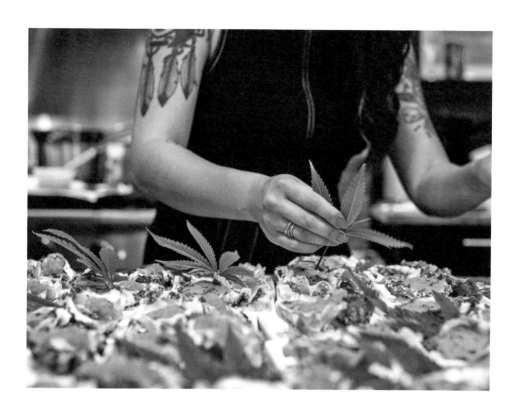

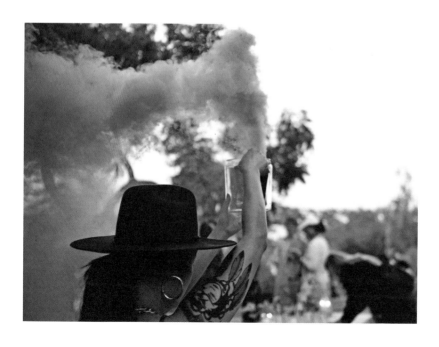

BIG BAD WOLF

A PERPETUALLY SOLD-OUT SERIES OF EXPERIENTIAL INFUSED DINNERS PREPARED BY KOREAN AMERICAN CHEF HAEJIN CHUN.

Haejin Chun loves cannabis, but that's not where she gets her high. I believe what really gets this effervescent founder and chef lifted is gathering her community with good food and cannabis and watching people find their tribe. Yes, her dinners include delicious, creative dishes influenced by her Korean family, the Mexican cuisine she loved while growing up in Southern California, and a two-year stint in Paris after college. However, what makes a Big Bad Wolf event is all the other personal touches: a seating chart organized for genuine connections and a custom playlist that complements the venue, occasion, and theme of the event. Sometimes Chun herself strolls past the tables with a colored fog machine to transport the guests to a different reality entirely. She understands the ephemeral, magical quality of a pop-up experience and how, when executed with love, those experiences can foster connections and inspiration long after the last bite of her signature black sesame dessert mochi.

Chun's experience in the cannabis realm landed her a consulting job on the Discovery+ show *Chopped 420* in 2021, and she continues to work as a cannabis consultant for the Food Network today. Until you're able to make it to one of her incredible dinners, you can make a little of your own Big Bad Wolf magic at home with *The Official High Times Baking Cookbook*, which she co-authored with fellow cannabis culinary leader Jamie Evans (www.theherbsomm.com).

Follow @bigbadwolfsf on Instagram for event schedule

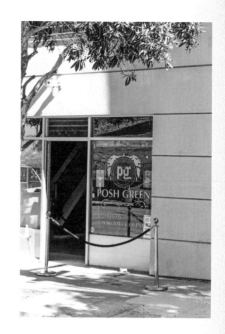

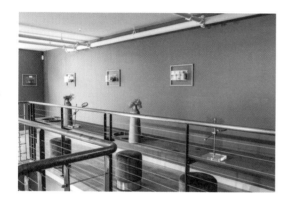

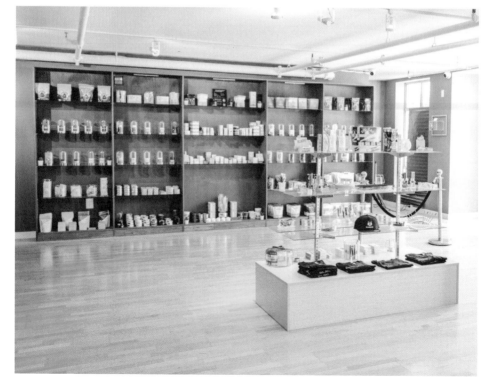

POSH GREEN CANNABIS

WOC-OWNED DISPENSARY WITH ALL THE SOPHISTICATION AND NONE OF THE PRETENTION.

Fancy aesthetics don't always equal quality experiences, but after spending many years picking up bud from a scrubby dude while carefully avoiding the laundry piles on his couch, I appreciate visiting a more polished environment every now and then. At Posh Green, you get a posh environment and extensive product offerings, all at accessible prices. It also happens to be the first shop independently owned by a woman of color to receive a license through San Francisco's equity program, which Posh Green founder and San Francisco native Reese Benton fought for by working with the city to advocate for policies that ensured minorities had a presence and a voice in this new industry.

With her elegantly furnished store, Benton aims to give every customer a luxurious experience, whether you are new to cannabis, medicating for relief and healing, or partaking for recreation.

There's a great variety of cannabis products on Posh Green's well-designed shelves, from Potli Dream Honey—made with nothing but raw wildflower honey and a 2:1:1 ratio of CBN, CBD, and THC to complement your bedtime tea—to Pure Beauty's sustainably grown indoor flower and pre-rolls in their chic, colorful packaging. There are also fun accessories in stock, like bejeweled glass joint holders.

Open Monday–Saturday

**828 Innes Avenue, Suite 110
San Francisco, CA 94124**

poshgreencollective.com

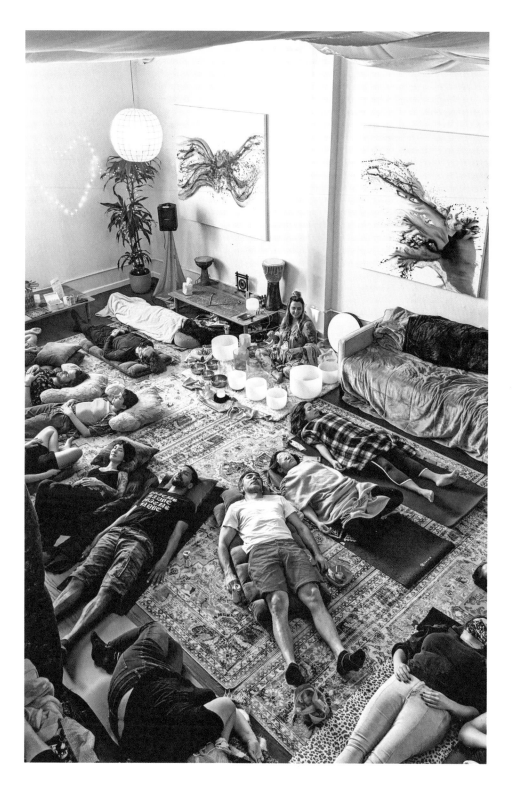

NOUERA

CANNABIS WELLNESS EVENTS LED BY SPIRITUALLY CONSCIOUS, MINDFULNESS-BASED ASIAN AMERICAN CO-FOUNDERS.

Since 2017, the impacts of the women behind Nouera have been seen and felt throughout the Bay Area, whether locals know it or not. In 2022, they helped produce the first cannabis retail and consumption lounge, Jardin de Hierba Buena, at the city's annual Carnaval festival, and in their daily business, they aim to cater to more casual consumers with their Smallz pre-rolls, which come in a variety of manageable sizes. In addition, Nouera puts on regular BYOC consumption-friendly sound bath sessions in Berkeley and San Francisco that include traditional tea ceremonies led by co-founders Cynthia Boedihardjo and Jessica Sharp. The first hour of the sound bath is dedicated to the educational tea service, during which attendees learn about cannabis and how it interacts with their bodies as they sip.

"I believe the use of cannabis helps people sense the energies and feelings moving through their body, allowing them to more easily tap into their intuition centers," Boedihardjo said. "Cannabis heightens the attendees' ability to focus on the sound being played and that which may be hindering them from getting where they want to go."

Once everyone has partaken in their preferred manner, guests are invited to head to the studio for a sound meditation journey via instruments ranging from crystal bowls and chimes to a *shruti* box, ocean drum, and mouth harp.

For event schedule, visit nouera.co

ROSE MARY JANE

AN OAKLAND-OWNED INDUSTRY FAVORITE FOR PICKING UP WELL-CURATED GOODS NEAR LAKE MERRITT.

Originally founded by Oakland resident Erik Murray, Rose Mary Jane busts a lot of myths about the cannabis retail game. It proves that you can make spaces that are beautiful and inspiring, that real talk about social justice issues can coexist with a chic canna-beverage bar, that you don't have to abandon your community to go bi-coastal, and that you can find success by stocking your shelves with small, locally owned brands. The folks over at Rose Mary also have an answer for anyone questioning their standards, with their strict vetting system for products—coined Rose Mary Jane Certified™—which requires that products meet or exceed state quality and safety standards and that employees and cannabis plants are treated with the utmost respect. Over 30 percent of the brands Rose Mary Jane carries are equity-owned cultivators and manufacturers, with most of them being from Oakland, including Smoke Champs and Happy Trails.

The Oakland location is a licensed cannabis consumption space, but unfortunately, you can't smoke there. Only cannabis edibles and beverages are allowed to be consumed on the premises. *What's the point of that?* you might ask. For this dispensary, it's about the principle of equal access to cannabis and safe spaces to consume it. You see, the law in California—and in many other states—really only permits consumption in private residences and licensed consumption lounges. If you rent, it's up to the landlord's discretion. If you reside in federally subsidized housing, consuming cannabis on the premises is altogether banned because it's still federally illegal. So on one hand, RMJ's lounge is indeed a chill place to sip a weed drink, partake in edibles, and socialize. And on the other, it's a statement about the illogical, inequitable way state and local governments are regulating consumption laws.

Open Daily

2340 Harrison Street
Oakland CA 94610

SUNSET PIPELINE

A TRUSTED DISPENSARY REGULARLY STOCKED WITH THE FINEST BAY AREA—GROWN INDOOR FLOWER.

This is one of the industry's favorite shops, or at least it's where my friends tell me they shop when they're doing canna-business in San Francisco. Sunset Pipeline's modest space is stylish but not stuffy, with a modern design, tons of natural light, and plentiful transaction stations for swift service during a rush. It's where you can typically find local THC heroes like SF Roots, the city's first equity-licensed farm and cultivator of absolutely fire flower, as well as Auntie Aloha's mouthwatering passionfruit-orange-guava gummies (my go-to for a tasty, tropical-flavored alternative to an anti-anxiety pill). There's an impressive cannabis beverage section here, too, offering a range of fast-acting options for those seeking an efficient high dose or a controlled small one.

Everything on the shelves is stocked with intention, reflecting quality, diversity of ownership, and a larger selection of Black-owned brands than many stores in the city. Regulars enjoy that there's always something fresh and new to try, while newbies will be relieved that the staff is prepared to help them navigate the broad menu for exactly the kind of cannabis experience they seek.

Open Daily

2161 Irving Street
San Francisco, CA 94122

sunsetpipeline.com

AMBER SENTER, CANNABIS ADVOCATE AND FOUNDER OF MAKR HOUSE

makr.house

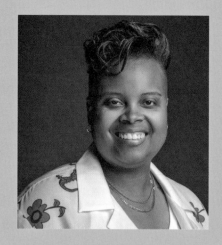

MAKR House founder Amber Senter is one of the biggest names in the fight for a diverse cannabis industry in California, as well as one of the most personally influential people I've interviewed over the years. I first encountered Senter while she was advocating for equity in cannabis at Oakland City Hall as a co-founding member of Supernova Women, a nonprofit empowering more people of color to become shareholders in the industry. Alongside fellow co-founders Nina Parks and Sunshine Lencho, their grassroots efforts helped pass Oakland's social equity program and reduce the heavy tax burden on licensed operators in the state, as cannabis businesses cannot benefit from many of the business expense deductions that every other business can.

Between ongoing efforts with Supernova Women and meetings with key legislators like California congresswoman Barbara Lee, Senate Majority Leader Chuck Schumer, and Senator Cory Booker about the challenges of well-meaning cannabis business owners, Senter runs MAKR House, a brand house that aims to build inclusive supply chains from the ground up and create more opportunities for entrepreneurs to successfully enter the cannabis industry.

HOW WOULD YOU DESCRIBE THE CURRENT TEMPERATURE OF THE CANNABIS INDUSTRY IN OAKLAND AND THE BROADER BAY AREA?

There are a lot of people that are not around anymore—some we miss and some we don't. I am encouraged by the headlines of major publicly funded companies, like Curaleaf, pulling out of California. I'm like, "That's right, they are! Because of people like me, and I'm proud." It shows that money isn't enough if they aren't going to include us—as in Black and Brown and queer folks, and small craft operators who care. We are the sauce; this industry is built on creative, craft operators.

WHAT ARE THE BRANDS UNDER THE MAKR HOUSE NAME RIGHT NOW?

Landrace Origins is a coffee and cannabis company featuring beans from a women-run farm in the Congo that are roasted locally by my cousin and paired with specific strains in store. It's about honoring the tradition of the wake-and-bake as well as demonstrating the possibilities of an inclusive supply chain: the complementary flower pre-rolls that accompany the beans come from special small farms like the woman-owned Ghost Ranch Dance.

Disco Jays are joints that are infused with THC diamonds (high, potent, THC concentrate that looks like crystals) on the inside and outside, so it's a visibly glittery joint—a real disco stick. But I also saw an opportunity to tell a story about the influence of queer, Black, and Brown communities on culture in general. I'm a queer Black woman born and raised in Chicago, who grew up listening to Chicago house music and going to house shows. Queer people were also at the forefront of legitimizing cannabis as medicine, and I want people to know that these communities are a big part of cannabis culture and pop culture in general. This is a pre-roll you take to a party *and* a pre-roll with a message.

WHAT BROUGHT YOU TO THE NOVEL BUSINESS MODEL OF MAKR HOUSE?

This whole brand house concept has been flying under the radar, but it's the lowest barrier of entry into cannabis. Both our brands work with the Equity Trade Network for distribution, which includes a printing company; the Disco Jays manufacturer is a longtime colleague and a longtime small business advocate who primarily employs people of color. We all work together to uplift each other.

So few independent entrepreneurs can afford the extremely high costs of getting their own licensed space with the right zoning, commercial kitchen abilities, production infrastructure, etc., and this offers an alternative avenue toward starting a business of one's own in the cannabis industry without taking on the full liability of being a licensee. It's a bit tougher to manage because you have to build a network you trust and the margins can be slim, but I think it's a business model that many could and should explore.

WHAT'S YOUR ADVICE FOR ASPIRING ENTREPRENEURS WHO ARE FIGHTING TO LOWER BARRIERS OF ENTRY INTO THE CANNABIS INDUSTRY IN OTHER CITIES AND STATES?

Culminate a strong small business community. Small businesses are the biggest employer in the US. They're more sustainable for the environment, they use less resources, and they keep the money in the community. Learn what can make it more possible for them to succeed and prioritize their needs from the start, and an inclusive, level playing field will naturally follow. Women, the queer community, people of color—a high tide lifts all boats. Be thoughtful, use critical thinking, and, if there's one thing to take away, vote with your dollar.

ROSE LOS ANGELES

A THOUGHTFUL EDIBLE BRAND TAKING A GOURMET APPROACH TO FRUITS, VEGETABLES, AND SUNGROWN CANNABIS ROSIN.

If you're looking for gummies in the state of California and you also care about the quality and flavor of every single ingredient, there is one brand I recommend: Rose Los Angeles (or Rose New York, if you're shopping in New York). The brand takes a farm-to-table approach with their signature Rose Delights, from the fruits and vegetables sourced for flavor to the fresh-pressed flower rosin used to infuse each gummy cube.

The original Rose Delight was a true spin on a Turkish Delight, infused with cannabis rosin grown under the sun at their farm in Penn Valley, CA, flavored with an organic rose hydrosol and layered with organic hibiscus flower. Alongside year-round offerings—both in dispensaries and online—they make seasonal batches like Ground Cherry Cola, a Delight made with ground cherries from their farm and a house-made, eight-ingredient cola syrup blend of piloncillo, citrus, nutmeg, coriander, vanilla, and their Gush Mints flower. They also make Rose Caps, a pure CBD extract made with flower rosin from their farm.

Founders Nathan Cozzolino and Scott Barry opted for flower rosin as their infusion ingredient because of its whole-bodied potency. Their high production standards for all of their ingredients has helped destigmatize edibles in gourmet foodie circles, and their support of small, often family-operated Emerald Triangle farmers is helping to fairly compensate the growers doing things the old way, with care.

roselosangeles.com

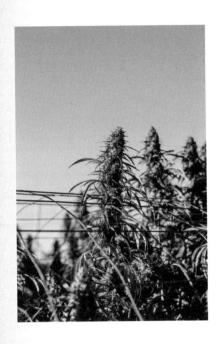

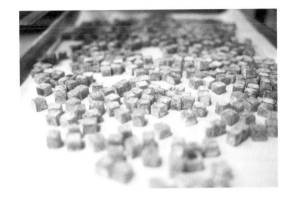

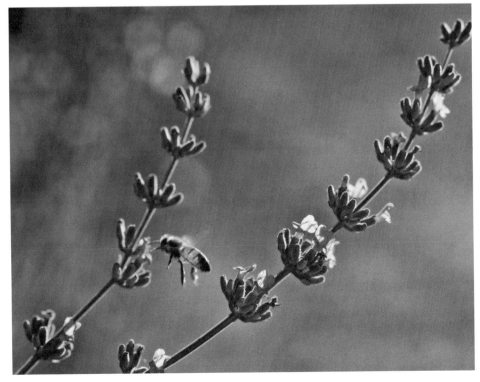

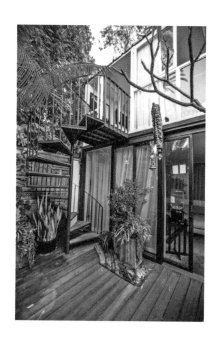

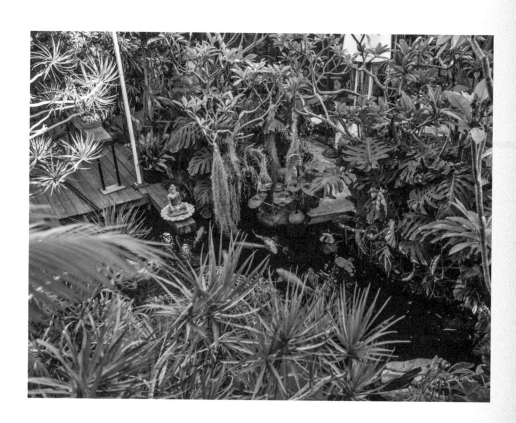

THE WOODS

A DISPENSARY AND OUTDOOR CONSUMPTION LOUNGE LOCATED IN A LUXURIOUS PRIVATE GARDEN RETREAT.

The California cannabis scene is awash with celebrity-founded ventures, but no amount of fame or money guarantees a project that actually turns out. Does anybody know what happened to Justin Bieber's cannabis line? Anyway, The Woods, cofounded by Woody Harrelson and Bill Maher, is impressive and undoubtedly here to stay.

The open-air consumption lounge is attached to a dispensary and situated within an incredible garden oasis, where resident parrots perch on lush, leafy branches and koi fish swim past Buddha statues in ponds. This stunning secret garden was formerly the private courtyard of the Schoos Design studio. The parrots—Lilly, Molly, Rio, and George—were owned by the studio, but Woody and his team suggested they stay in their familiar home, free to experience a new chapter of this botanical paradise. The flora and fauna simply transport you, like taking an overnight flight and waking up in Thailand. Plus there's a good chance for a celeb sighting. Last time a friend visited, they said their night included accidentally slamming Jon Hamm with a bathroom door and accidentally calling Owen Wilson by his brother's name, Luke.

Each of The Woods' private, rentable cabanas are totally unique, interesting structures, with one at the heart of the property being a ten-by-ten-foot, all-glass cube with white curtains and another being accessible via a spiral staircase into the tree canopy. Smoking is only allowed in the designated smoking structures, but you can freely consume edibles and enjoy non-infused tea or hot cocoa from the still-evolving tonic bar. The novelty and sheer beauty of this space has kept it a major destination in the Hollywood neighborhood, and because there's nowhere quite like it, there's a good chance you'll see one of the owners popping in for a "work meeting."

Open Daily

8271 Santa Monica Boulevard West Hollywood, CA 90046

thewoodsweho.com

GORILLA RX WELLNESS

A WOMAN-OWNED DISPENSARY DOING GOOD FOR DIVERSE ENTREPRENEURS AND THE SOUTH CENTRAL NEIGHBORHOOD.

The first Los Angeles dispensary opened by a Black woman also happens to also be one of the finest in the city, a South Central gem that's coursing with the energy of the community that got it going. Founder Kika Keith was well known long before Gorilla RX Wellness opened its doors for her work assisting other aspiring entrepreneurs in completing the complicated application process for social equity licenses. Keith's detailed records while doing this work ended up serving as evidence that the city illegally accepted a number of licenses before the official time window for the public began. This eventually led to the city allowing an additional one hundred social equity licenses to be issued—a huge victory in a state with a low number of licenses allowed in many cities—the first of which was Gorilla RX Wellness.

Standing a mere eight blocks from where Keith grew up, her bright, welcoming shop is a warm introduction to legal cannabis for anyone. It's a worthy stop for connoisseurs seeking out a well-curated menu of minority-owned farms as well as newbies looking for edibles in a broad range of flavors and potencies. If you want to start small, I recommend a ten-milligram seltzer to sip on or a fresa con crema chocolate bar from La Familia.

Open Daily

**4233 S Crenshaw Boulevard
Los Angeles, CA 90008**

gorillarxwellness.com

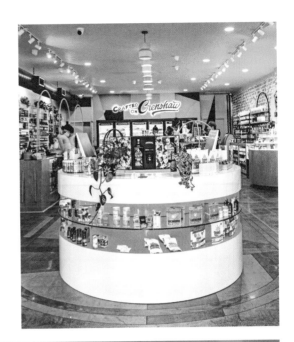

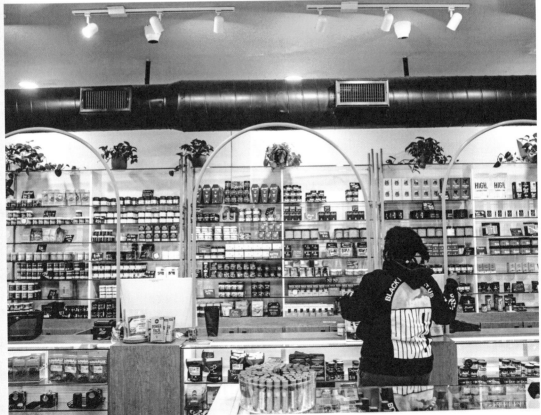

HIGHLITES

A SERIES OF WELLNESS EVENTS AND YOGA WORKSHOPS DESIGNED TO HELP ONE REWRITE THEIR RELATIONSHIP WITH CANNABIS.

Despite being a fifth-generation Japanese American, I was born into a fairly cannabis-friendly West Coast family that didn't subscribe to the same serious stigma around the plant that many other immigrants have. As I had more conversations over the years with people from different backgrounds, I learned that I'm a bit of an exception, so I love the work Highlites is doing to bring a compassionate, creative, and healing safe space to people of all backgrounds while supporting the cannabis-curious with group yoga and meditation sessions.

When founder Danielle Olivarez initially started Highlites in 2018, she was hoping to meet like-minded women who loved cannabis and yoga. Once she discovered this community was in need of connection and guidance, the certified yoga and meditation teacher with a background in Tibetan Buddhist meditation started hosting classes and events that welcomed consumption, but in a more mild and very intentional way. Over time, the classes grew into what Olivarez calls an "oasis of stoners who care." Highlites is more than a consumption-friendly space; it's a safe space to microdose cannabis, move, and grow together.

For event schedule, visit highlitesoasis.com

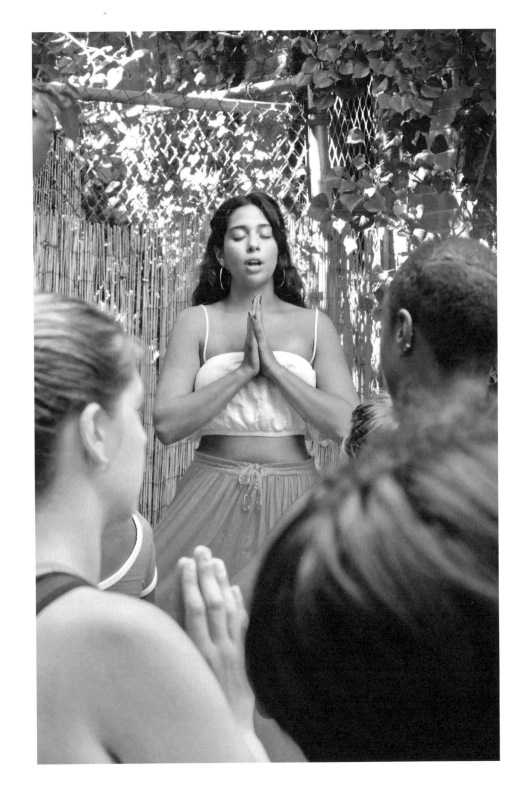

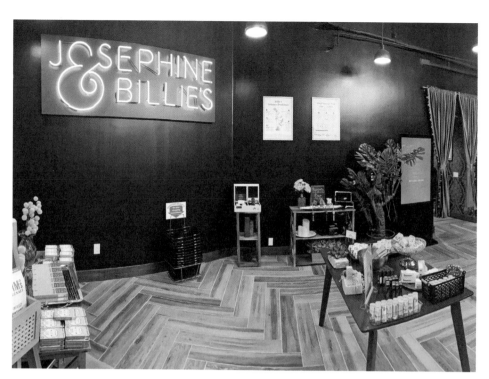

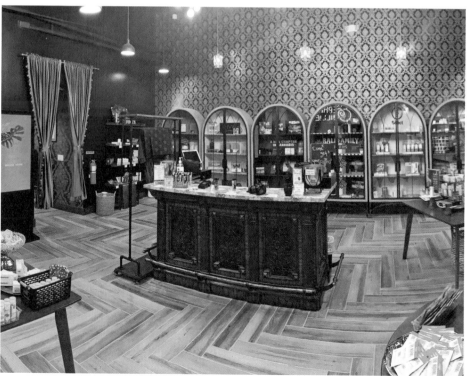

JOSEPHINE & BILLIE'S

A BLACK-OWNED, FLOWER-FRIENDLY SPEAKEASY PAYING HOMAGE TO BLACK MUSICIANS OF YESTERYEAR.

In the 1920s and '30s, when stars like Josephine Baker and Billie Holiday were headlining marquees, there were semi-secret safe spaces for Black and Brown communities to be merry and smoke a little reefer, known then as "teapads." For co-founders Ebony McGee Andersen and Whitney Beatty, the history lesson is as important as plant education, and their considerations for the cannabis-centric needs of marginalized communities are reflected throughout the aesthetic décor of Josephine & Billie's.

Both Andersen and Beatty discovered the medicinal benefits of cannabis following anxiety attacks. Cannabis changed their lives and inspired them to not only change their careers, but also their own stigmas around the plant. Beatty grew up in the 1980s on what was known as the "most dangerous street in the country" in Detroit, Michigan, witnessing the violence inflicted on communities in the name of the War on Drugs. As a child and into adulthood, cannabis scared her, but once she learned what it could do for her mental and physical state, she went back—way back—to understand why the government had been so hard on this ancient herb. She learned how normalized medical cannabis was prior to the 1920s and how politicians like Harry Anslinger intentionally spread a false narrative that aligned it with Black and Latino communities in a negative way. So, this period-themed dispensary goes beyond the decor to rewrite that negative narrative around cannabis.

From the moment you walk in, J & B's invites you to revisit the past and this plant with fresh eyes, honoring the cultural legacy of jazz, Black artists, and cannabis itself while presenting the weed in a pleasing, medicinal manner. Instead of a scientific series of glass vials for terpene education, there's a charming lineup of old-fashioned perfume bottles for guests to peruse. The flower selection is rich with product from minority-owned farms like Ball Family Farms and Stone Road Farms, and it's organized with a more nuanced potency rating system that gets you much closer to finding your desired effects than the oversimplified binary of sativa and indica. Beatty and Andersen hope to make space for women who, like them, needed to see cannabis in a different light.

Open Daily

1535 W Martin Luther King Jr. Boulevard Los Angeles, CA 90062

josephineandbillies.com

MISTER GREEN LIFE STORE

A LEADING CANNABIS-CENTRIC BOUTIQUE SELLING STREETWEAR, HOME GOODS, ART, AND SMOKING ACCESSORIES.

Self-described as a "friendly shop for high-minded people," this low-key boutique has led the charge of cool, cannabis-adjacent offerings since 2015. I wrote about the shop's blend of mind-altering art, 1960s relics, and super modern, artisan-made smoking paraphernalia in the debut issue of *Broccoli* before I even knew the founder and old-school hippie Ariel Stark-Benz was a fellow Oregonian. The career designer has a portfolio that includes Nike and Ace Hotel, but these days, he's the embodiment of Mister Green, seeking out international craftspeople to collaborate on thoughtful, utilitarian, and beautiful creations, from Italian leather stash bags to branded grow bags for backyard pot grows. Countercultural impulses come naturally to him, and his eye for wit and craft have led to creations like the Bong Water Nalgene—a patented, tongue-in-cheek water bottle labeled with the last thing you'd ever want to drink. This interest in referencing the old and the new is also reflected in the featured pieces by other artists, like the apple-shaped ceramic pipes by Summerland and the beautifully bound Lune Noire notebooks that feature hidden compartments for storing smoking tools.

But more than a hip destination, Mister Green's goods speak to the weed-friendly version of the hiker-skater-surfer fantasy with sincere authenticity. Stark-Benz's hemp goods collection was inspired by his lifelong search for the perfect, 100 percent hemp Oxford shirt for a few reasons: hemp feels and looks great, it's one of humanity's earliest known textiles, it's more biodegradable than cotton, and its crops require less water while absorbing more CO_2 than cotton crops. In 2023, Stark-Benz opened a second location in Tokyo, Japan, where he lived for a time, providing what I imagine is a very meaningful hub for a community that's only known a highly stigmatized social climate around cannabis.

Open Daily

**3019 Rowena Avenue
Los Angeles, CA 90039**

For more locations, visit green-mister.com

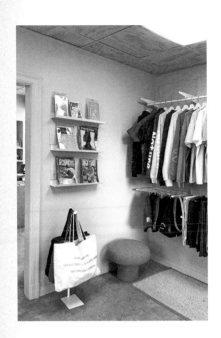

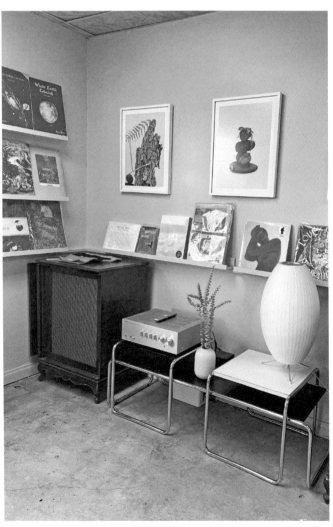

THE ARTIST TREE

A LIVELY, MULTISTORY DISPENSARY AND LOUNGE FILLED WITH UNIQUE ART AND ACTIVITIES.

Every one of the Artist Tree locations are unique, artful spaces that make shopping for weed an adventure of its own, but the West Hollywood location—complete with an art gallery and a well-appointed indoor/outdoor consumption lounge—stands above the rest. All artwork on display at the stylish store is for sale directly by the artists, and the consumption lounge is designed like the living room of a mansion you'd admire in a magazine. Well-stocked bookshelves line the rich, dark blue walls, and there's a variety of seating that can be reserved ahead of time, including the airy, romantically lit patio. Although guests are not allowed to bring their own cannabis from home, they're able to smoke or order edibles to munch on, and there's a tasty, non-infused food menu available throughout the day.

Luckily, you don't have to purchase anything if you want to just check the place out, but why not grab a pre-roll from Seth Rogen's Houseplant or HUMO, a brand celebrating Latin pride. There's a variety of accessories available for complimentary use or to rent, or you can bring papers from home. If you're into the scene but not the smoke, The Artist Tree has got you covered there too, with their designated non-smoking area on the third floor reserved for non-combustible consumption. Every type of consumer deserves a space to kick back with fellow cannabis lovers. You might even find your non-consuming friends tagging along for a visit, whether they're down to join you for one of the weekend yoga classes, a speed dating sesh, or a burlesque show.

Open Daily

**8625 Santa Monica Boulevard
West Hollywood, CA 90069**

For more locations, visit theartisttree.com

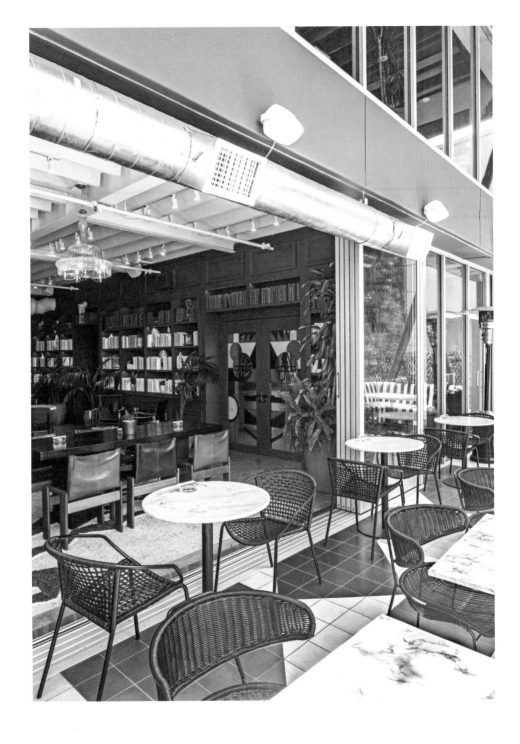

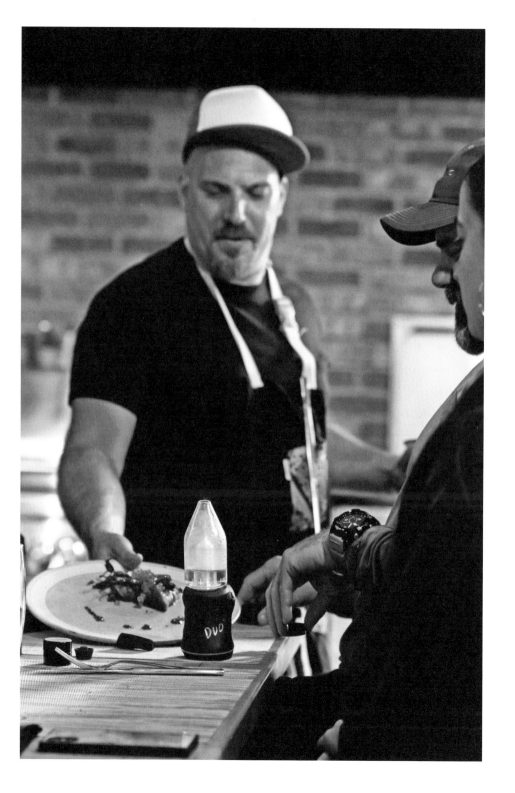

CANNABIS SUPPER CLUB

A CANNABIS-INFUSED FINE DINING SERIES COMPLETE WITH CHEF TASTINGS AND WINE PAIRINGS.

I relate to Cannabis Supper Club founder Marc Leibel's fascination for cannabis. He enjoys it, he wants to help others expand their understanding of it, and he likes good food, but he does not have the culinary prowess to combine those pursuits. Same, TBH. Instead of attempting to fit a square peg into a round hole, Leibel tapped Chef Chris Binotto—featured on Netflix's 2020 cannabis-infused culinary show *Cooked With Cannabis*—to develop a monthly multicourse dinner series that pairs dishes with curated cannabis strains. Binotto was inspired by the opportunity to craft such multisensory experiences and eagerly joined as executive chef. Leibel and Binotto consider the flavor of the flower as well as its effects when deciding what strain best complements which dish, often pairing appetizers with more energetic strains, like mushroom crostini and Beyond Blueberry flower from Wonderbrett, and meat dishes with heavier strains like OG Kush.

Eating infused food is a very different experience from smoking while you eat. Sometimes I want to eat as much as I want without worrying about getting uncomfortably high. Cannabis Supper Club understands this and offers guests the chance to enjoy food to any degree they'd like.

"Wine pairing has been going on for how many years now—how many years of science and research and experience," founder Marc Leibel said. "Sometimes it's really complementary, and a perfect match of strain and food bring out one another's flavors in interesting ways. And sometimes, it's just smoking some great weed while eating some great food."

For event schedule, visit cannabissupperclub.com

LAPCG

A LONG-ESTABLISHED DISPENSARY WITH A MEDICAL LEGACY AND STERLING REPUTATION FOR WELL-SOURCED PRODUCT.

A pattern has emerged in many states, in which, following adult-use legalization, the medical market is left by the wayside. There is more money to be made on the recreational side with more potential customers, but it's the medical side that made all of this possible. The medical growers and dispensaries advocated for legal cannabis to exist and showed state regulators that those of us dealing in cannabis can be trusted to be professionals. My first cannabis industry job was budtending at a medical shop, and it was incredibly special to serve customers who talked about the life-changing impact cannabis products had on their lives. Despite most shops flipping to recreational once the laws evolved, those patients still go to the same dispensaries and are still dealing with serious ailments. Over the years, dispensaries have begun catering less and less to medical patients, and LAPCG is a glaring exception to that trend.

Short for "Los Angeles Patients & Caregivers Group" and established in 2004, LAPCG is one of the longest running dispensaries in the city, and it is as beloved by recreational customers now as it has been by medicinal patients for all these years. The budtenders are educated and experienced, not just in product recommendations but in listening, being patient, and answering questions.

Once inside, the calm, streamlined space makes for an efficient visit that won't overwhelm you with a lot of bells and whistles. They have a well-stocked menu, with plenty of the basics and many interesting, novel smokables like Drew Martin's mildly dosed cannabis pre-rolls that include herbs like lavender and passionflower. They also carry one of my all-time favorite edibles: delicious, ginger-spiced, 5 mg THC and cardamom-rose-infused hard candies from Cosmic View.

Open Daily

**7213 Santa Monica Boulevard
West Hollywood, CA 90046**

lamedicalmarijuana.com

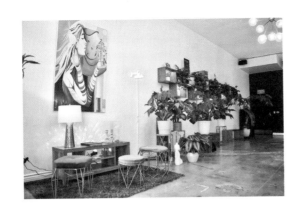

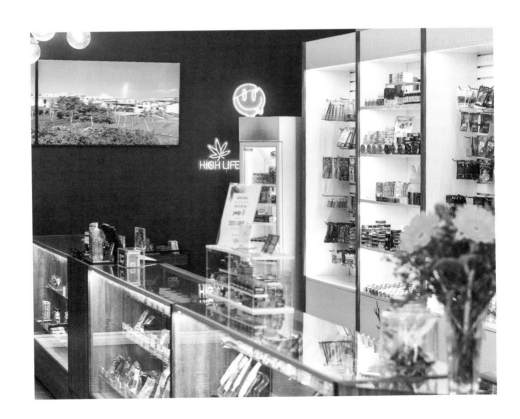

CHEF WENDY ZENG

PIONEERING CHEF BORN IN CHENGDU, CHINA, MAKING FARM-TO-TABLE INFUSED FARE IN EAST LA.

Since winning the Food Network's competitive cannabis cooking show *Chopped 420*, Chef Wendy Zeng has established herself in California's rich culinary cannabis scene with memorable dinners and collaborations that often honor the flavors and traditions of Chinese cuisine. She works with brands in and out of the cannabis industry through her company Drizzle Catering, but she has also partnered with community figures for one-of-a-kind events, like her work with cannabis-centric baker and writer Christina Wong on Mogu Magu, an event series inspired by Magu, the healing hemp goddess found throughout ancient Asian literature. You'll also see her collaborating with Cannabis Supper Club co-founder and chef Chris Binotto on live-fire dinners.

When I asked her about the most memorable dishes she's created in the past, she spoke of creations that allowed her to incorporate seasonal herbs and fruits from her garden.

"One of my favorites is my passionfruit scallop crudo garnished with spicy, fruity, and smoky peppers," Zeng said. "I also love cooking anything on a live fire. I've always been fascinated with fire as a kid, and now as a chef, I've learned to appreciate the transformation abilities to bring out textures and flavors."

Zeng regularly hosts chefs from around the world for cannabis-friendly dinners on her property in East Los Angeles. To her, there is no one dinner or experience that adequately captures all the joy cannabis can bring.

"My ultimate dream is for the space to host all kinds of cannabis culinary experiences that make people feel a sense of community and feel empowered in their consumption journey. If we want to destigmatize and have people accept cannabis, we have to make sure cannabis experiences make all kinds of people feel accepted."

Follow @wenyerhungry on Instagram for event schedule

drizzle.catering

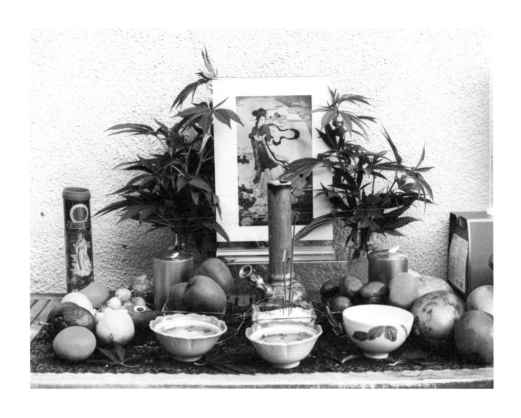

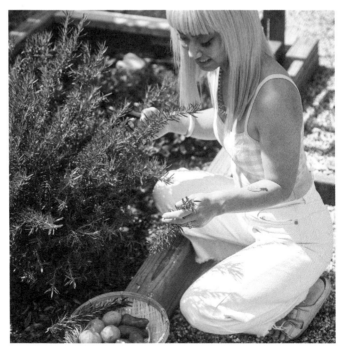

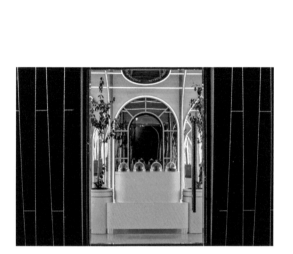
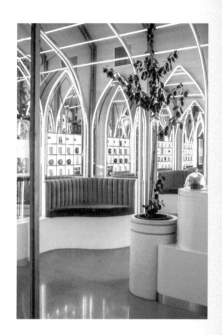
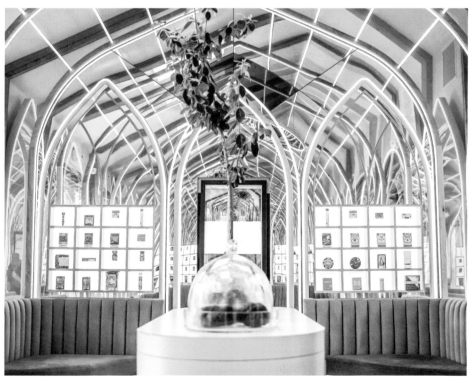

WYLLOW

USING LIGHT, COLOR, AND MIRRORS, THIS MICRO-DISPENSARY IS ANYTHING BUT SMALL, OFFERING A UNIQUE MENU AND A ONE-OF-A-KIND BUILDOUT.

There is a simple, reflective storefront along South Robertson Boulevard that, depending on the time of day, might have a slight neon glow emanating from its entrance. You might stop to take a selfie in the exterior's mirrored facade without realizing that you're standing in front of one of the most beautiful dispensaries in the world, both inside and out.

Entering WYLLOW is like walking into an immersive art exhibit, with its multicolored lights, mirrors, and iridescent glass magnifying the space into a magical chamber of light and color that can completely transform the vibe on a dime. The shop was founded by Camille Roistacher and her husband and business partner, Josh Roistacher, a pair of industry veterans who have successfully run a cannabis brand and distribution company since 2018. While the shop opened in 2021, the WYLLOW cannabis brand has been on shelves for a minute, offering flower by the eighth and a range of regular and oil-infused pre-rolls. They seek out unique cultivars you won't find just anywhere, grown by legacy partner farms with many years of experience. Everything in the shop, from the products to the overall design and decor—developed by Tina Fung of the design firm SpaceObjekt—was intentionally sourced to provide opportunities for potentially overlooked vendors.

"I've seen this industry from both sides," Camille explained. "I know how competitive it is to get shelf space in dispensaries, and I want this store to be a destination for women-owned brands, queer-owned brands, minority-owned brands—brands that deserve a chance to showcase their products but maybe haven't gotten the opportunity to do so. We hear from many vendors that we are their first stockist."

One of those indie finds Camille recommends are the delicious rosin-infused gummies by Oui'd, which, although founded by two Michelin-starred chefs, hadn't had luck landing any stockists before WYLLOW.

Open Daily

**2622 S Robertson Boulevard
Los Angeles, CA 90034**

shopwyllow.com

NEW RITUALS

A SERIES OF VIBEY, AESTHETICALLY CHIC, CONSUMPTION-FRIENDLY WELLNESS EXPERIENCES HOSTED ACROSS LOS ANGELES.

Stoned yoga is something I practice regularly alone, but group experiences never get old. It doesn't have to be fancy, and it usually isn't, but the wellness-oriented, yoga-centric classes put on by New Rituals are something else entirely.

After years of being the go-to person in her yoga community for all things cannabis, Lexi Kafkis decided to streamline her mindful cannabis recommendations and combine her two passions—yoga and weed—to create New Rituals, a cannabis-friendly wellness collective that facilitates classes and one-on-one coaching to empower people to rewrite their relationship with themselves, others, and the planet through cannabis. Live musicians are often involved in these intimate events, which typically host no more than fifteen people at a time and take place at creative spaces owned and operated by fellow cannabis believers.

To begin, each guest receives and enjoys a pre-roll from a sustainable, sungrown farm partner. Following the brief, low-dose smoke break, Kafkis guides attendees through a breathwork session to help them assimilate to the high. Then comes sixty minutes of slow-flow yoga, deep stretches, incense, and groovy music. Throughout the average class, Kafkis also shares the history of the plant and yoga alongside info on the body's endocannabinoid system, which at this point is fully activated.

In addition to this Smoke and Stretch event, New Rituals hosts sound baths, Cacao and Kush ceremonies, summertime forest-bathing excursions, and workshops on women's healthcare and cannabis based on Kafkis's personal experience using cannabis while living with endometriosis and polycystic ovary syndrome. This range of Rituals' events speaks to the wide array of reasons people call on cannabis to help deal with issues in their minds and bodies.

For event schedule, visit createnewrituals.com

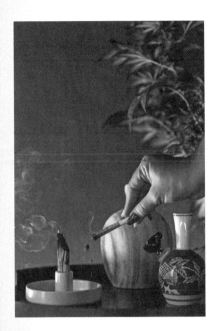

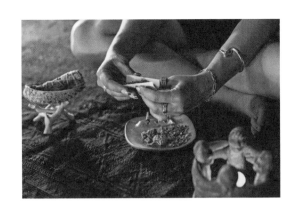

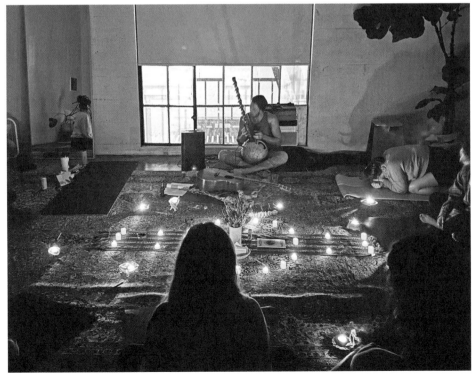

CORNERSTONE WELLNESS

AN INDUSTRY STAPLE FOR THOSE LOOKING FOR WELL-SOURCED, THOUGHTFULLY GROWN FLOWER IN LA.

If you ask someone who's worked in the LA weed scene for a recommendation of a legit shop, one run by people who care about the quality of their cannabis products, chances are they'll recommend Cornerstone Wellness. This shop is so well respected because, beyond intentionally sourcing for the menu, founder Erica Kay maintains relationships with the sungrown cultivators she sources her flower from, visiting ahead of harvest season most years. Her staff is also known for their cannabis-science savvy and patience.

For nine years, it was solely a medical shop, but since the state legalized recreational use, it's been a dual adult-use and medical shop. Many patients still come here to pick up, and many adult-use shoppers come for medicinal-leaning products. Regardless, all kinds of people come here because they trust that the products will be potent and come from producers they want to support. Every bud of flower and sip of cannabis beverage is stocked with the intention of supporting small, independent craft farms committed to sustainable and regenerative cultivation practices. As a first-generation Latina, Kay has also made sure Cornerstone Wellness prioritizes shelf space for fellow female, minority, and LGBTQIA+-owned cannabis brands.

Open Daily

**2551 Colorado Boulevard
Los Angeles, CA 90041**

cornerstonecollective.com

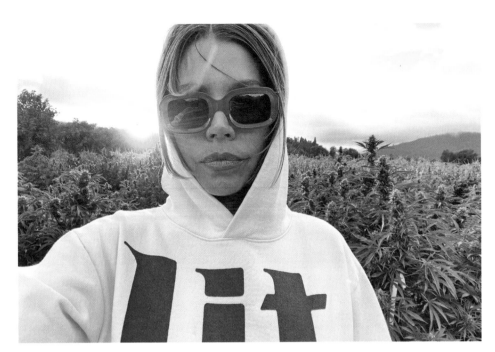
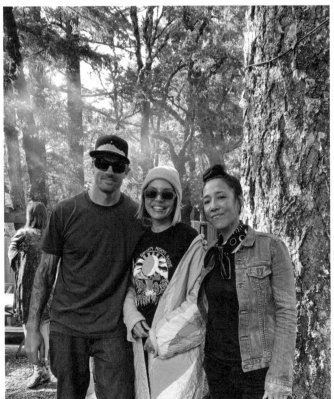

HICKSVILLE PINES CHALETS & MOTEL

QUIRKY, CANNABIS-FRIENDLY LODGING FEATURING THEMED ROOMS THAT CELEBRATE POP CULTURAL FIGURES.

There are places that try to be quirky, and then there are places crafted with such painstaking, particular care that they end up being quirky to anyone besides the founders. The Hicksville Pines Chalets & Motel, sitting about an hour's drive west from Palm Springs, falls into the latter category. A riff on the similarly kooky Hicksville Trailer Palace in Joshua Tree, this motel is heavily themed around many pop culture staples, including David Lynch's cult TV series *Twin Peaks*, with a suite named "The Great Northern" that's decorated like, well, the Great Northern Hotel from the series. That three-bedroom unit has velvet red curtain details and graphic floors to match scenes from the show, and guests can listen to the iconic soundtrack on vinyl while lounging by the fireplace.

While I am a *Twin Peaks* fan, you'll find me in the Dita, a private chalet retreat designed by the burlesque diva herself, Dita Von Teese, and her interior decorator, Stacia Dunnam. There's a round retro bed, a glittered two-person clawfoot tub, a bathroom fireplace (does it get more glamorous than that), and a grill guests can use on the private deck. It's a non-smoking unit, but you can consume cannabis outdoors in most areas of the property, and if you rent the 420 room, you can smoke indoors.

The 420 room is a 1970s-inspired space with psychedelic art on every wall and a sunken queen bed flush with the floor, perfect for when you hit the in-suite Volcano vaporizer so hard that you start worrying about falling off. This is considered the Rolls Royce of vaporizers, and one with which I've made many chill, giggly, and cough-free memories. The suite also includes a vending machine filled with snacks, a record player with a carefully curated selection of albums, wide-open mountain views, and a TV stocked with streaming platforms for your mellow, bingeing pleasure.

This motel also has a Dolly Parton-themed room and a John Waters-inspired "Mondo Trasho" suite that features a closet full of outfits in the spirit of his delightfully demented muse, Divine. You don't need to love weed to come here, but it's a joyous privilege to get to enjoy cannabis while you lodge.

23481 CA-243
Idyllwild-Pine Cove, CA 92549

hicksvillepines.com

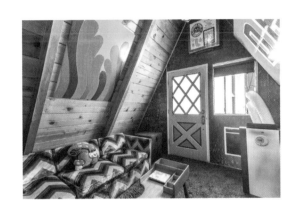

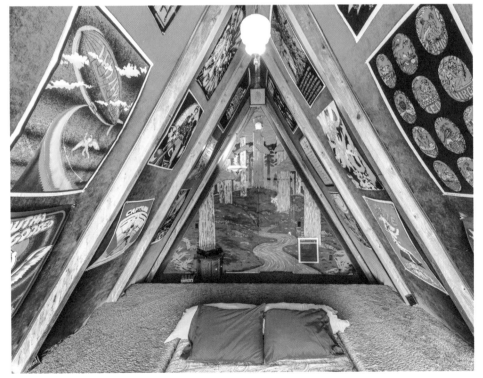

LIGHTHOUSE

MINIMALIST-CHIC DISPENSARIES STOCKING A BROAD SELECTION OF THE STATE'S FINEST BRANDS WITH LOTS OF LOCAL PRIDE.

This pair of chic, well-supplied shops in the Palm Springs area may appear to prioritize style, but Lighthouse is yet another example of a shop that cares about its community as much as its photogenic quality. There is room for spaces like these, especially in the broader effort to remove the stigma around buying and enjoying cannabis as a craft herb rather than an illegal drug. The Coachella shop looks like it's built inside of a refurbished air hangar, with a sloped metal roof that frames the sweet little cactus garden around its entrance. The spacious Palm Springs location includes a coffee counter and a consumption lounge. Beyond bougie surrounds, though, Lighthouse has worked to authentically welcome many parts of the community. Come Pride Season, co-owner Joseph Rubin and his team regularly host viewing parties on their patio to watch the parade go by (they've also hosted drag shows at the Palm Springs location), and they offer shuttle transportation to and from retirement facilities in the community.

Alongside flower, pre-rolls, and vapes aplenty, Lighthouse offers versatile options for low-dose edible experiences, like Kikoko's infused herbal teas, Papa & Barkley's THC capsules, and infused Cheeto-like cheesy chips by TSUMo Snacks. It's hard to eat just a handful of those THC-laden chips, so if you're looking for non-infused snacks—and happened to be headed to Joshua Tree—I recommend checking out the **Wine & Rock Shop**, a very cute indie market with all kinds of interesting handmade goods and artisanal bites you can binge.

Open Daily

**395 N Palm Canyon Drive
Palm Springs, CA 92262**

**For more locations, visit
lighthousedispensarypalmsprings.com**

Wine & Rock Shop

**59006 Twentynine Palms Highway
Yucca Valley, CA 92284**

TORREY HOLISTICS

A LONG-ESTABLISHED AND TRUSTED NEIGHBORHOOD SHOP PUTTING REGENERATIVE FARMING FIRST ON THEIR SHELVES.

This unassuming neighborhood shop in the Sorrento Valley neighborhood of San Diego was the first adult-use dispensary to be approved in the state of California. That proves a few things: they know what they're doing, and their menu and service has stood the test of time. They're also one of the first shops recommended to me by my San Diego-based weed writer colleague. Torrey Holistics' thoughtful selection of well-curated flower, edibles, dabbing/vaping oil, and more has kept it a local favorite by connoisseurs and first-timers alike. Devoted to both medical patients and recreational customers, the budtenders here are well-versed in the menu and are passionate about catering to each individual's needs. Bonus points for their menu prominently stocking and featuring Sun+Earth Certified flower, which you can trust will deliver pure, potent effects.

In the community, Torrey Holistics has partnered with the nonprofit Feeding Kids First for the past six years to host in-store food drives for children experiencing food insecurity within San Diego county.

Open Daily

10671 Roselle Street, Suite #100 San Diego, CA 92121

torreyholistics.com

NG APOTHECARY HERB SHOP & TEA BAR

ALSO KNOWN AS THE CHURCH OF HERBALISM, THIS HERBAL APOTHECARY HOSTS CANNABIS-FRIENDLY EVENTS IN BARRIO LOGAN.

Nayeli Gutierrez first started formulating herbal tinctures to help her family members with health issues ranging from anxiety and body aches to diaper rashes and sore throats. As more family and friends saw positive results from her products, she got more interested in the magic of herbs and became a certified Holistic Health Practitioner. She started selling her tinctures at pop-ups and farmers' markets, eventually making a home for NG Apothecary at her Logan Avenue storefront.

What this physical retail space has grown into is much more than just an herb shoppe; it's the Church of Herbalism. Head through the front door painted with whimsical, winding vines and find a haven for herbally minded folks, with rows of carefully sourced plants, herbs, and spices for patrons to choose from. In one trip, you can pick up nontoxic bug repellent made with lemongrass, tea tree, and eucalyptus essential oils; smokable hemp and herb joints; and hand-poured beeswax candles with flower petals and healing crystals embedded in the surface.

Beyond the tinctures and herbal blends, Gutierrez carefully sources hemp clones (clippings) so people can grow their own at home. She also opens the space for cannabis consumption-friendly events, ranging from art showcases and sip-and-stitch sewing tea parties to candle-making workshops and free sound therapy sessions.

"It's very powerful hosting cannabis events that are women-centered because a lot of these ladies are solo stoners," Gutierrez said. "It fills me with so much giddiness to see the look on their faces when there's a whole room of thirty-five to forty-five like-minded women all smoking weed together. It's amazing to be able to connect both of these herbal industries in our own way because, at the end of the day, cannabis is a flower, and we love flowers."

Open Wednesday–Sunday

**2205 Logan Avenue
San Diego, CA 92113**

ngapothecary.com

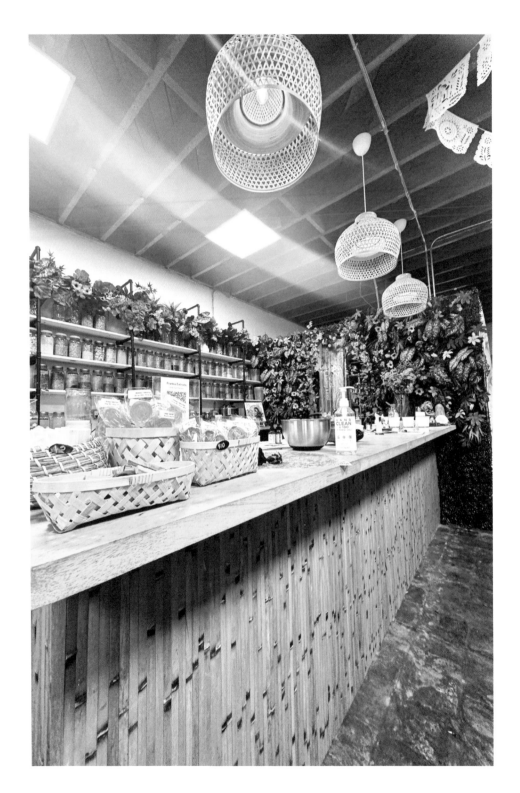

MARCH AND ASH

A DISPENSARY CHAIN KNOWN FOR ITS BEAUTIFUL, PLANT-INSPIRED SPACES AND EXPANSIVE SELECTIONS.

March and Ash is the kind of place where locals take visiting relatives so they can "ooh" and "aah" at the impressive-ness of New Weed. Each location is clean, organized, and beautiful, with a playful interior design that references familiar words and imagery from decades of cannabis culture. More than that, though, March and Ash is consistent and trustworthy. It's a place that locals know will provide the contemporary cannabis shopping experience they're looking for, the kind of experience one seeks when heading to a Whole Foods or New Seasons, for example. This is how it should feel to purchase legal cannabis—like you're in qualified, grown-up hands.

The exact menu items at each location slightly differ depending on availability, but sought-after farms like Pure Beauty, a cool brand I've interviewed multiple times over the years for their radical approach to sustainability (they have their own wind turbine on the roof of their indoor grow!), and Farmer and the Felon, a brand founded by a longtime cultivator who served six and a half years in prison pre-legalization, are always in stock. The shop's name is a nod to the founders' belief that cannabis can play a beneficial role in our life cycle, with March symbolizing the start of spring and new life, and Ash representing a life lived and fertilizer for new beginnings. I also find it special that when you shop here, you're supporting workers that have successfully unionized with the United Food and Commercial Workers. In 2021, the company agreed to a contract agreement granting employees wage guarantees, profit-sharing, and a $30,000 annual contribution from March and Ash to cover their childcare and education expenses.

Open Daily

2835 Camino del Rio S #100
San Diego, CA 92108

For more locations, visit
marchandash.com

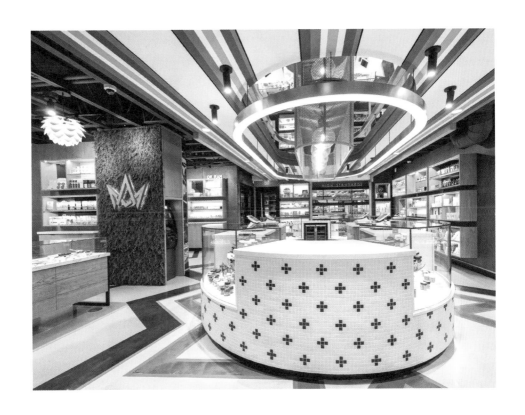

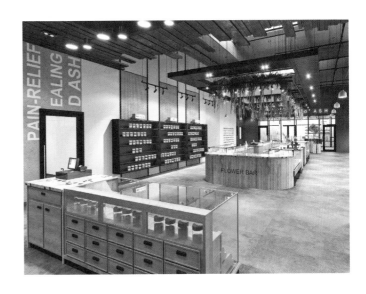

With a city culture that celebrates artisanal crafts and farm-to-table fare, my home base of Portland, Oregon, was destined to be a unique cannabis hotspot as soon as the state legalized. Accessible licensing processes lead to more dispensaries here per capita than anywhere else—two hundred in Portland alone, more than the number of McDonald's locations statewide. For consumers, it's an affordable playground of some of the most strictly tested and seriously vetted legal cannabis grown in the country. Based on my biased adventures down the West Coast and around Amsterdam and back, the best cannabis in the world is cultivated in this humble, low-ego community of science-forward growers, many of whom were key in building my network of trusted sources and mentors. You won't find an ample selection of consumption lounges in Oregon, but certain Portland hotels—*cough* the Jupiter Hotel *cough*—quietly feature smoking-friendly outdoor areas. What the City of Roses lacks in big city offerings, it more than makes up for with its sprawling offerings of city parks, homegrown cafes, and globally renowned dining destinations, all of which wouldn't bat an eye if you showed up in jeans and Birkenstocks.

Although it's often referred to as "eastern Oregon," Bend is really smack dab in the middle of the state, the last larger city before the mostly remote, desert-y expanse between there and Idaho. A high-altitude destination for skiers, hikers, and fans of independent breweries, it's a rapidly growing city with a no-frills, outdoors-oriented vibe. The increasingly poppin' music scene draws in major musical headliners throughout the year, and it's very normal to smell cannabis at any given concert. There is a small airport that flies direct, or it's a three-hour drive from Portland, which does allow for a satisfying stop at the stunning Smith Rock State Park to stretch your legs.

PORTLAND

BEND

PORTLAND

ORE

LEGALIZED

Medical in 1998,
recreational in 2014

POSSESSION

Adults over the age
of twenty-one can
possess: one ounce
of cannabis flower,
five grams of extracts,
and more edibles than
you could possibly
consume in one day.

HOME GROWS

You can buy up to ten
cannabis seeds and grow
four cannabis plants
at home.

DELIVERY

Yes, but only to private
residences (no hotels).

CONSUMPTION

Smoking is allowed
on private property,
but in natural spaces
throughout the city, you'll
often smell respectful
consumption happening
somewhere out of sight.

CITIES

Portland
Bend

BEND

PORTLAND

BEND

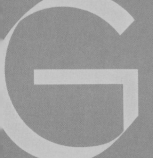
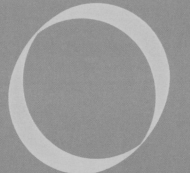
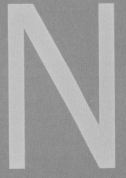

CAREFREE CANNABIS

A RELIABLY CHILL NEIGHBORHOOD DISPENSARY OPERATED BY MY FAVORITE GROWER IN THE PNW.

When I first started my cannabis writing career, one of my first strain reviews was for Cherry Kush grown by a farm called Nelson & Co. Organics. It was operated by Greg Levine, who named it after his beloved pet spaniel and catered specifically to medical patients, which meant he needed to serve a certain number of patients in order to expand his grow with more plants. I hit it off with the Illinois expat and became one of his patients, benefitting from an ounce a month of his incredibly rich, glittering buds, all grown from old-school genetics he'd gathered over the past few decades. I came to deeply admire his painstaking, reverent approach to growing cannabis, never getting swept up by trends or hot new competitors.

When he and his cultivation partner, Mike Ciarlo, got licensed in the recreational program and I let my medical registration lapse, I continued to follow their flower around town. And when they started flash-freezing fresh flower and sending it to the renowned processors at Pua Extractions, who then used chemical-free, ice water methods to create flavorful, strain-specific hash rosin, me and every other connoisseur in town chased that around, too.

They are quiet members of Portland's scene compared to the brands paying for billboards and flashy sponsorships, but if you ask any grower who's been around since the medical days, they have nothing but respect for Nelson & Co.'s products and indoor cultivation practices. As Levine and Ciarlo still do almost everything themselves, they don't have aspirations of a grand expansion or multistate presence. They want to do things their way, ensuring that their flower and concentrates are always as good as they can be. And since they've stayed small, their flower moves quickly whenever a dispensary receives a Nelson & Co. drop. So you can imagine how excited I was when the pair co-founded their very own spot, Carefree Cannabis, ensuring a home base that's always stocked with some of the Pacific Northwest's—if not the entire West Coast's—finest flower and hash goods.

Open Daily

**5926 NE Killingsworth Street
Portland, OR 97218**

carefreepdx.com

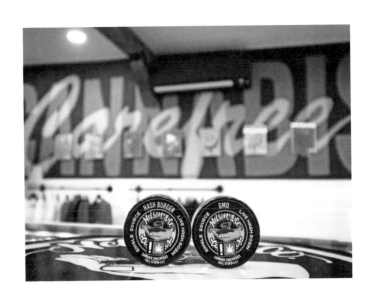

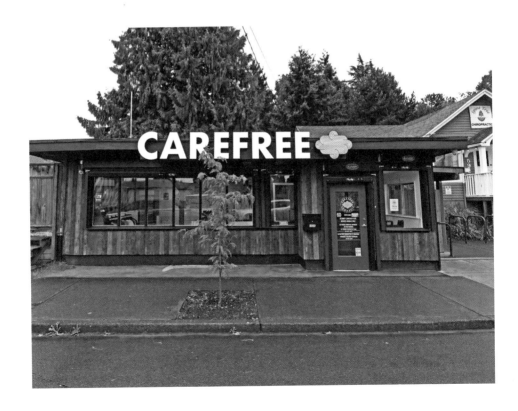

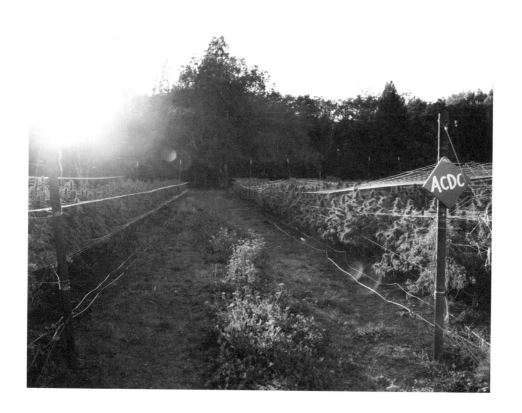

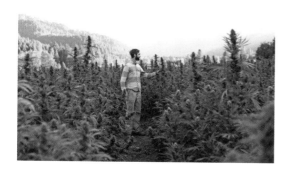

EAST FORK CULTIVARS

A TRUSTED, FAMILY-RUN HEMP FARM WORKING TO MAKE THE CANNABIS INDUSTRY HEALTHIER AND MORE ETHICAL.

There is only one farm that comes to mind when folks talk about CBD in Oregon, and that's East Fork Cultivars. Founders Nathan and Aaron Howard planted their first licensed crop in 2015 with the goal of growing the best CBD-rich cannabis possible, and from where I'm standing, that's exactly what they've been doing ever since. East Fork is so legit that they are licensed in Oregon's adult-use weed program so they can sell high-quality hemp without being restricted by the >0.3% THC rule that defines hemp on a federal level. In recent years, they've even invested extra time in identifying CBD-rich strains after seeing their brother, Wesley Howard, experience fewer symptoms from his medical conditions.

To say their sungrown flower is grown with care would be an understatement. In 2018, East Fork was one of the first hemp farms to be certified organic by the USDA. Most Oregon dispensaries mentioned in this book sell a strain or three from East Fork—in flower, pre-roll, or tincture form or inside many of the CBD-leaning edibles on the shelves.

eastforkcultivars.com

GREEN MUSE

THE WORLD'S FIRST HIP-HOP DISPENSARY, CELEBRATING BLACK CULTURE AND COMMUNITY IN NORTHEAST PORTLAND.

Green Muse is touted as "the world's first hip-hop dispensary," and that identity is reflected in more than just the graffiti murals inside and '90s rap playing in the background. Initially going by the name Green Hop, the shop is the creation of co-founders Karanja Crews and Nicole Kennedy, both Portland natives and former educators who were interested in honoring the legacy of Black culture in cannabis as well as in this part of Northeast Portland. Up until this neighborhood was gentrified in the 2010s, it was a predominantly Black community for decades, one that dealt with neglect and increased targeting from police. Today, it's virtually unrecognizable from the Woodlawn neighborhood that Kennedy remembers, with its new trendy cafes, upscale restaurants, and shiny apartments too expensive for former neighborhood residents to rent.

Green Muse stands on one of the last Black-owned lots in the neighborhood, and in that regard, it's working to balance the rapid change of gentrification, creating space for Black Portlanders to feel like they still belong.

Located in a brightly colored converted Craftsman home, Green Muse is a bastion for all cannabis lovers wandering the area. Inside, the colorful space is all personality, with classic records from artists like De La Soul and A Tribe Called Quest on rotation and hip hop-inspired art covering the walls. The flower selection is as solid as the vibe, with a great selection of affordable buds as well as primo offerings from sought-after names like the beloved inner-city farm LUVLI—don't miss their Leftovers strain if it's in stock—and the sustainable soil savants at Green Source Gardens. If you're going the gummy route, don't miss Astral Treats' full-spectrum, strain-specific gummies. The effects will be slightly more predictable knowing what individual strain it's infused with, and the signature star shape makes it easy to divvy up into smaller doses.

Open Daily

**5515 NE 16th Avenue
Portland, OR 97211**

greenmusecannabis.com

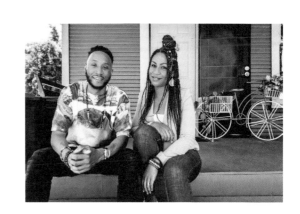

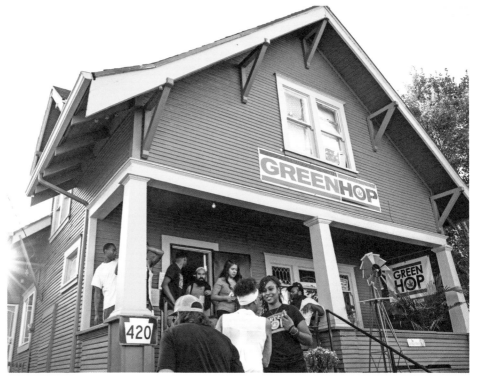

MAKE AND MARY

A CBD BOUTIQUE OFFERING HOUSE-MADE SKINCARE AND BEAUTY PRODUCTS AS WELL AS ARTISAN CRAFT WORKSHOPS.

Founder Yvonne Perez Emerson took the concept of "everything is more fun when you're high" to a whole new artistic level when she launched her weed-infused workshops and art classes in 2016. Emerson is a familiar face in Portland's art community, and one of my favorites from past interviews. Her warm, curious nature is infectious, reflected in the diverse spread of artists, healers, and spiritual practitioners that have enthusiastically accepted an invite to lead a Make and Mary session. These heritage craft workshops have included everything from macrame and leather work to floral crown-making and sound bath sessions cushioned with an infused tea ceremony. At each event, attendees are welcome to bring their own product or enjoy provided potables, and the consumption is more of a side bonus than the focus of these gatherings. It's about giving creatives the whimsical off-time they require as much as providing a welcoming entry point for crafty cannabis newbies (and a fun date for people who'd rather get stoned than buzzed).

These events take place at Make and Mary's brick-and-mortar—which Emerson runs with her daughter—seated at the start of the Green Mile of dispensaries along Portland's NE Sandy Boulevard. Outside of the events, Emerson has tapped into her lifelong relationship with plant medicine to craft a house line of CBD-infused beauty and wellness products. I'm a fan of the calendula face mist and hand-poured scented candles myself. Informed by recipes handed down and inspired by her Mexican and Scottish heritage, the soothing serums and moisturizers, flattering cheek tints, and CBD-infused bath bombs are made to nourish the skin with only the most essential, carefully sourced ingredients. The shop is a bit of a wellness retreat in itself, with lots of plants and a comfortable, spa-like atmosphere that invites you in with a refreshing "ahh."

Open Tuesday–Saturday

2506 NE Sandy Boulevard
Portland, OR 97232

makeandmary.com

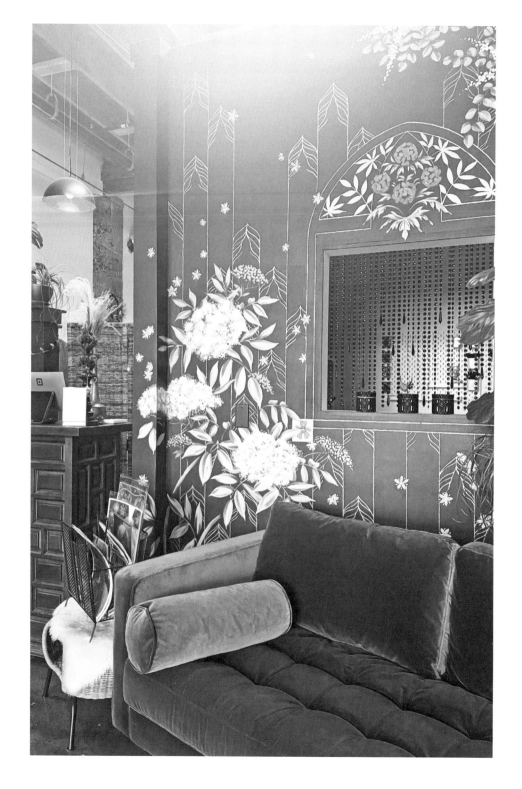

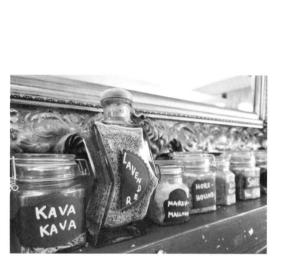

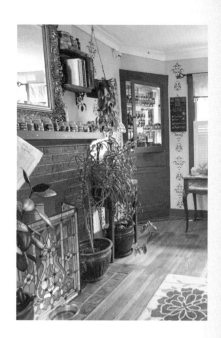

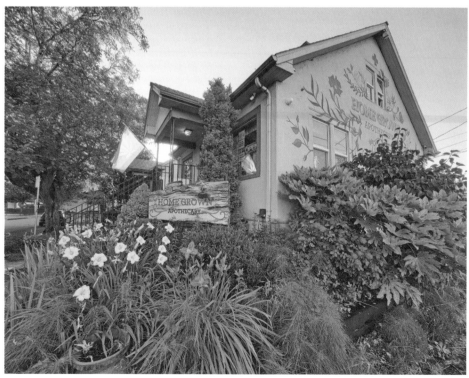

HOME GROWN APOTHECARY

A CHARMING NEIGHBORHOOD DISPENSARY SELLING A VARIETY OF HERBS, PLANTS, AND CAREFULLY SOURCED FLOWER.

Herbal remedies take on new meaning here, where loose-leaf calendula, marshmallow root, elderflower, and cannabis are ethically sourced, heavily vetted, and sold by the ounce. Founder Randa Shahin, a former professional snowboarder, focuses on supporting minority-owned, woman-owned, LGBTQ+-owned, and family-owned farms, but that's only the start. She only considers stocking flower that was grown in real soil, without chemicals, on farms with serious sustainability goals. The edibles must be infused with product that meets those same flower standards, and they can't contain any artificial flavors or irresponsibly sourced palm oil. Additionally, cartridges and vape pens must be made free of filler oils and artificial flavors.

In a town where many share Shahin's values, that still leaves a solid selection for Home Grown Apothecary's patrons. Green Source Gardens and Utokia are a couple of the farms regularly on rotation, as well as respected concentrate processors like Sun God Medicinals, the maker of an RSO tincture that, when consumed in a tiny, pearl-sized amount daily for a few weeks, helped my friend's weird nerve issue in their dominant arm disappear entirely (definitely still consult your doctor for any health issues you may be having). There are also cannabis plant starts for sale, skincare products formulated by the in-house herbalist, and non-cannabis smoking herbs to help folks quit tobacco. The charming converted residence feels exactly the way a cozy, independently owned herb shoppe should: welcoming, healing, and a little magical.

Open Daily

**1937 NE Pacific Street
Portland, OR 97232**

homegrownapothecary.com

NOMSTERNAILZ

A CREATIVE, CANNABIS-FRIENDLY NAIL ARTIST WHO IS HAPPY TO FACILITATE A SESH AS YOUR SET DRIES.

My good friend Nomi Miraj has always loved the soothing, creative ritual of getting high and doing her nails, although she didn't pick up the habit until she moved to the West Coast from Gwanju, South Korea, in her youth. Miraj ended up in Portland to study graphic design, eventually graduating from Portland Community College. Soon after, though, the challenging financial prospects of being a young designer starting out in a competitive design scene became clear, and she couldn't ignore the fact that she spent more money on beauty than design services every month. So, instead of waiting for a design project, she started offering nail services to her friends in 2018, ones that welcome cannabis consumption before, during, and after the treatment. Then she started offering to come to them, and Nomsternailz's mobile, weed-friendly nail salon was born.

Over the years, Miraj has popped up at all kinds of cannabis events with a limited selection of nail art services, expanded into her own physical space in Northwest Portland's Alphabet District, and continues to offer home visits for a modest fee. She is always happy to accommodate requests and design references for nail designs, but, if you let her, she will freehand some incredibly artful and totally original nail art. When I booked her for a vacation mani ahead of a trip to Japan, she painted little detailed cherry blossom branches, Hokusai waves, and a *maneki-neko* (the "beckoning cat" you see at the front of many businesses) on different nails. Korean nail culture is wildly more adventurous. Miraj has pointed out to me that it's totally normal for conservative business executives to have colorful, bejeweled manicures dangling with charms and Swarovski crystals, and she hopes to make space for that kind of boundless creative expression in Portland.

To book a service, visit nomsternailz.com

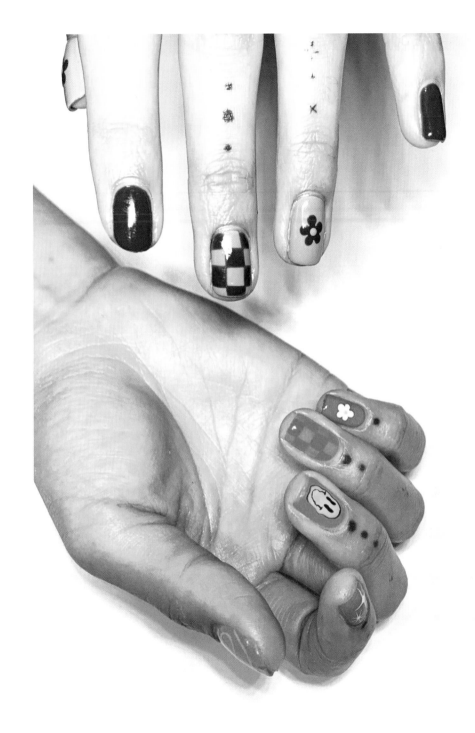

SOMEWHERE

A SOPHISTICATED DISPENSARY IN THE NOB HILL NEIGHBORHOOD SELLING PLANTS OF THE SMOKABLE AND NON-SMOKABLE VARIETY.

When it's time to restock on any kind of greenery, Somewhere is a particularly peaceful stop. Its big windows make it feel like you're stepping into an actual greenhouse—not to mention the dozens of potted plants and starts filling nearly half the store's interior. More interested in that baby monstera than an eighth of flower? That's OK; the budtenders are just as helpful when navigating which plant would thrive best in one's low-light apartment. You can browse anthurium starts and potted cacti, carnivorous plants, and wandering philodendrons, all priced as affordably—if not more so—than any other plant store in town. Hand-blended teas by local brand T Project can also be found on the shelves.

Founders Oliver Garnier and Luke Rodgers hope their thoughtful curation of various goods from the natural world can help "reestablish the dialogue between flora and humans," presenting cannabis alongside tea leaves and exotic plant leaves to take it out of the drug realm and remind people that it is also a plant. Rather than packing their shelves with interchangeable brands, they prefer to prioritize quality over quantity. On any given day, there are only a handful of strains on the menu; the founding team prides themselves on a "zero filler" menu, only carrying flower in its freshest state. Every time I visit, I discover an interesting strain I haven't seen at other popular shops, and it's always freshly cured.

Somewhere carries a range of cartridges, plus trusted all-in-one pens like the Quill, which measures and stops each inhale for an accurate and consistent low dose. On the edible side, you can find local bean-to-bar chocolate maker Leif Goods, whose 1:1 Mint Hibiscus Chocolate Bar has delivered balanced highs across the state for years. Somewhere also hosts a gardening workshop in the spring, offering free grow kits and in-person expertise to help people grow their own cannabis.

Open Daily

**2128 NW Overton Street
Portland, OR 97210**

somewherepdx.com

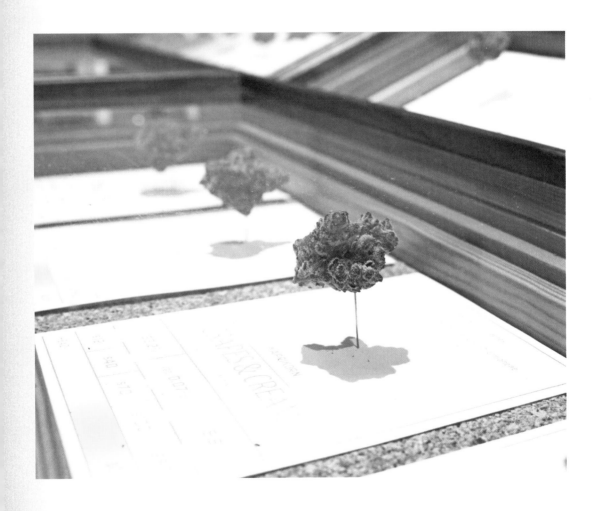

LIV VASQUEZ, CANNABIS CHEF AND PLANT MEDICINE EDUCATOR

livviesmalls.com

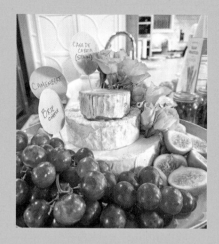

Numerous cannabis-infused supper clubs and dining experiences have come and gone since Oregon legalized cannabis, but Portland-based chef Liv Vasquez has stood the test of time, winning an episode of Netflix's *Cooked With Cannabis* along the way. This success can likely be attributed to her versatility as a lifelong student of plant medicine and a former employee in New York's restaurant industry. Vasquez currently offers one-on-one coaching on how to customize plant medicine, helps brands formulate new CBD products, teaches virtual cooking classes, and hosts catering events. Her events are experiential and educational, leaving guests with a full belly, a perfect dose of cannabis, and a better understanding of how this plant interacts with their bodies. I spoke with Vasquez about her favorite past events and what she loves most about Portland's cannabis scene.

WHAT WAS YOUR FIRST INFUSED CULINARY EVENT LIKE?

I moved to Oregon right when cannabis was legalized and totally shifted careers from the restaurant industry to cannabis, getting a job at a dispensary to learn everything I could. I had been cooking with cannabis for a long time, but I treated this like a DIY master's in cannabis. Three years into working in the industry, around 2018, I hosted a small infused brunch for mostly cannabis industry people. By that point, I had learned about absorption rates, infusing food with cannabis, endocannabinoid systems, and I wanted people to learn something here. Everyone was so happy throughout that brunch—it gave me the encouragement to keep going.

When LA decriminalized cannabis shortly after, I was like, 'Time to plant my flag there, too.' I found a building with a roof I could transform, and I pretty much constructed a restaurant on that rooftop for a whole experience. Built a kitchen, set up heaters, timed everything with the sunset, and offered the same scientific education to the guests.

WHAT ARE SOME OF YOUR FAVORITE EVENTS YOU'VE DONE OVER THE YEARS?

The caterings always surprise me. I'm working on an elopement next to a waterfall in Vermont right now. It's always an adventure, like you're putting together a big puzzle, and at the end of it, the guests are mesmerized because they get a whole experience—an experience that they really didn't know they could have. One that stands out in my mind required us to hike into a remote mountaintop. We had to meet this group of old friends where they were camping, which meant building and breaking down a whole dining table. We brought cannabis pairings and accessories to complement each course. This was a group that got together annually to honor a passed friend and celebrate life, and they all sat around the table smoking joints and sharing stories after. I'm so grateful I get to give those experiences to people.

HOW WOULD YOU DESCRIBE PORTLAND'S WEED SCENE?

I didn't know much about cultivation before I moved here. I'm from New York, where you don't know where your food grows, you don't know where your weed grows, you just have "a guy." Just as I was excited to go to farmers' markets and take control of my food supply chain, I love being able to do that here. I got into understanding the cultivation side, and there is such fascinating innovation and sustainable practices happening here. I moved here because of the food scene in Portland. It was known as a restaurant-driven town, a foodie town, and for ethical practices and good worker benefits in its craft culture, and that philosophy extends to many cannabis producers here.

WHAT FARMS/BRANDS DO YOU LOOK FOR WHEN SHOPPING?

I love Magic Hour for their great flower and how they operate and represent as BIPOC in the space. Same with LOWD. They don't miss; I try every strain of theirs. East Fork, for their founder story, their desire to make good medicine and treat their people well, their ongoing work advocating for legislative progress at the capital, and their beautiful hemp. I love everything they do. I also love Greater Goods CBD chocolates and sweets, House of Spain CBD topicals and tinctures, and Hapy Kitchen gummies—good people and good THC product.

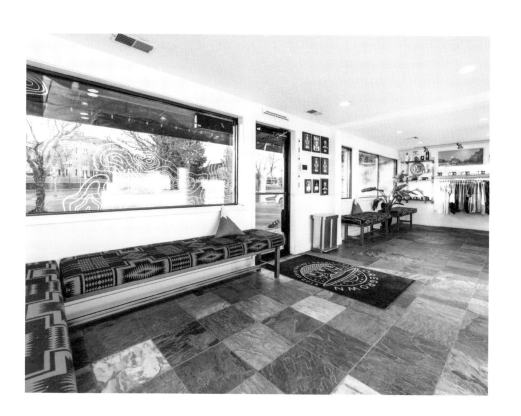

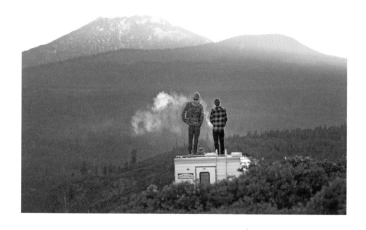

OREGROWN

A LONG-ESTABLISHED LOCAL CHAIN FOUNDED BY OUTDOORSPEOPLE, FOR OUTDOORSPEOPLE AND ALL WHO LOVE GREAT FLOWER.

Before cannabis was legalized for adult use, Oregrown was a beautifully branded medical cannabis farm and dispensary with well-designed, outdoor-oriented merch you'd actually want to wear. Today, it's a statewide chain that's remained a local favorite in Bend and beyond, with increasingly slick locations that make first timers feel at ease in a professional space. Longtime consumers will be satisfied by the range of fresh, absolutely fire flower on hand, highlighting many of the state's finest farms.

Oregrown grows house flower as well, which is priced strain-by-strain from $6–$15/gram to accommodate a range of pockets. Eugreen, Evan's Creek, and Focus North Gardens are other premium farms regularly stocked on these shelves that connoisseurs ought not miss. Edibles and concentrates are also well represented, from solventless passion-orange-guava gummies that give a full-bodied high to Altoid-like, low-dose options perfect for subtle consumption.

Although the founding team of Aviv and Christina Hadar and Kevin Hogan care about quality Oregon cannabis, the soul of Oregrown was born in the mountains of Bend, reflected by the imagery of their logo, the branded camping gear sold in the shop, and special side projects in the community like Low Pressure, a documentary they sponsored that showcased talented backcountry snowboarders exploring volcanoes, burned forests, and mountain ranges across Oregon.

Open Daily

1199 NW Wall Street
Bend, OR 97703

For more locations, visit
oregrown.com

TOKYO STARFISH'S BUD AND BREAKFAST

CHILL AND SPACIOUS CONSUMPTION-FRIENDLY LODGING ABOVE A POPULAR BEND DISPENSARY.

This vacation rental sits on top of the Westside location of Tokyo Starfish, a local chain of dispensaries offering a centrally located, consumption-friendly home base stocked with everything you'd need for a successful smoke sesh. The provided smoking accessories are stored in a locked case, which comes in handy for the surprising number of families that have stayed at this spot. That might have more to do with it being a two-bedroom with an additional futon in the loft, a full kitchen, and an ample balcony in a town where spacious accommodations get booked fast. But it also says something about shifting norms and the professional, comfortable environment around and above the shop.

In any case, this listing is regularly booked out, but that's not because it includes free product. There's actually no cannabis included in the rental, but you get a discount at the dispensary downstairs and you can smoke anywhere in the unit or on the balcony. It's also in a fantastic location: the Old Bend neighborhood at the heart of town, where you can stroll past century-old historical homes on your way to Jackson's Corner for the best casual brunch in town. You won't have to walk through the dispensary to get in and out every time—there's a private entrance—and while you may catch an occasional whiff of the shop, the unit won't smell like weed unless you're actively consuming some. Besides that locked case of smoking paraphernalia, a single bean bag in the living room is the only dead giveaway that this is a place built by and for people who love to smoke cannabis.

**542 NW Arizona Avenue
Bend, OR 97703**

tokyostarfish.com/bud-and-breakfast

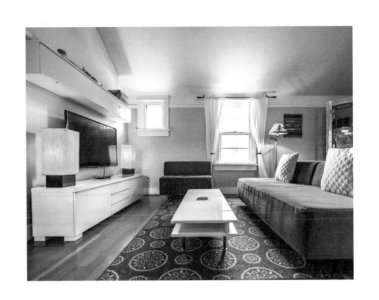

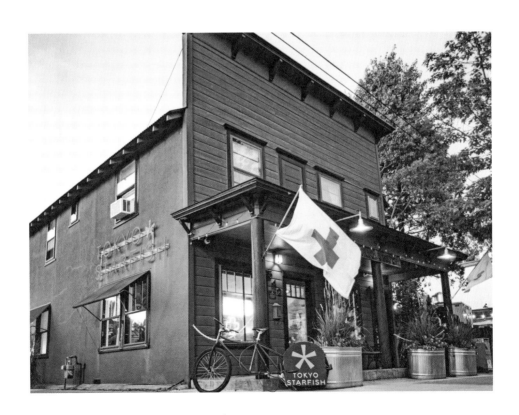

MAGIC NUMBER

AN EXPERIMENTAL INFUSED-BEVERAGE BRAND BORN FROM BEND'S RENOWNED CRAFT BREWERY SCENE.

Cannabis beverages are an exciting new part of the edible realm today, but, whew, let me tell you—the first generation of drinkable weed did not go down very smoothly. The cannabis extract would gather at the surface or the sides of the can, resulting in wildly inconsistent doses and really funky-tasting drinks. Magic Number was among the first to crack the code on formulations that kept the product evenly incorporated and tasty going down, and they're absolutely the first to make an infused sparkling cider in the state (packaged in a 750 ml bottle like the iconic Martinelli's apple juice, no less).

Since 2015, their range of beverages includes sparkling peach tea, classic cola, lime seltzer, and spicy ginger beer, each uniquely infused with live resin. This is a kind of cannabis concentrate created with heat and pressure, so no harsh solvents are used to remove the good stuff from the plant material, and more of that good stuff is retained in the final product.

People report a richer high, rounded out with the additional compounds besides THC that occur naturally in cannabis. With beverages, that high can be more easily dosed than, say, cutting a gummy into quarters, and the effects can be felt more quickly than the hour to hour and a half that edibles can take to digest.

Like many Bend residents, friends Dan Pilver and Alex Berger were experimenting with home brewing when the idea for Magic Number first germinated. Pilver, a special ed teacher by day, was developing his own ginger beer as a creative outlet after work, which led to their first product: a cannabis-infused ginger beer. They used recycled brewing supplies and called on friends to help with hand-filling bottles at first, eventually outgrowing Berger's garage and relocating to a real facility with industrial brewing capacities.

drinkmagicnumber.com

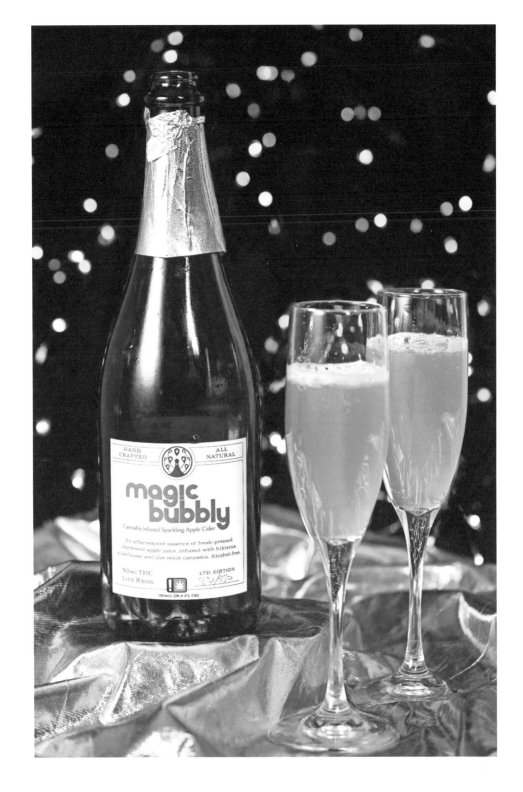

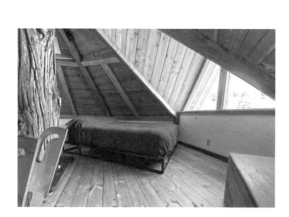

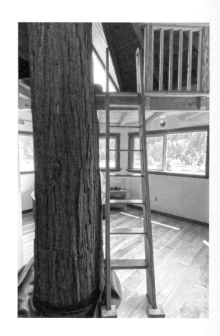

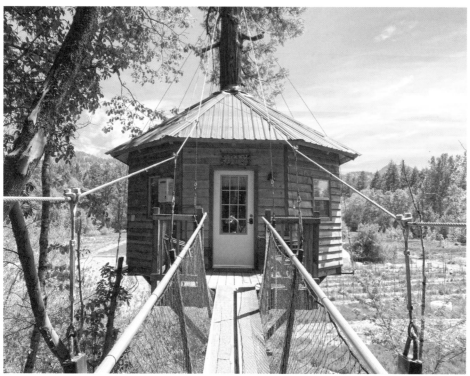

THE TOKINTREE HOUSE AIRBNB

CANNABIS-FRIENDLY, TARZAN-STYLE LODGING IN CAVE JUNCTION, OREGON.

Hours away from Portland and Bend lies a spacious treehouse perched above a cannabis farm. Located just a couple miles from the California border in the small town of Cave Junction, the TokinTree House is an off-shoot of the Out 'n' About Treehouse Treesort where breakfast and "activitrees" are available daily in a hippie paradise of quirky, roomy treetop abodes (plus one boat). This cannabis consumption-friendly rental is indeed located within a licensed cannabis farm, so all guests must be at least twenty-one years or older to stay. The treehouse accommodates up to four people, and since it is truly built into the canopy and branches of a tree, thirty-five feet off of the ground, that occupancy limit is not flexible. If it gets windy, it is possible there will be some creaks and movement, which is totally normal, but if it gets too hazardous, guests are moved into ground-floor units.

A complementary cannabis gift is guaranteed, and a garden tour is available, but not guaranteed. After all, TokinTree House sits on a working medical farm, and the folks here are sometimes too busy with the plants to accommodate a tour. Other licensed adult-use farms border the property—par for the course in this remote part of the state where the summers are long and hot. My recommendation if you find yourself visiting from September to November: Enjoy the plants from afar and let the team get to it. It's harvest season, and they've got trimming to do.

420treehouses.com

When Washington's adult-use stores first opened, I couldn't resist driving across the border for the experience. I had my medical card at the time, but it still felt special to just walk into a store with my sister like we were grabbing a bottle of wine. The weed was pre-packaged in a jar with vibrant packaging, which was totally different from Oregon dispensaries, where flower is typically weighed out by the gram into uniform plastic containers right in front of you. Today, I don't have to drive that far to pick up legal buds, but there remain plenty of reasons to head north into Washington's weed-friendly world.

The natural world reigns supreme in the Evergreen State, from near year-round skiing at Mt. Rainier to the many pristine lakes that draw Portlanders up every summer, not to mention some of the PNW's best concert lineups at the amphitheater perched above the Columbia Gorge—all of which lend thousands of opportunities for respectful consumption away from those who might be bothered. Despite Seattle's size, though, Washington's more cautious regulations have resulted in a much mellower cannabis scene in proportion to other West Coast states.

Throughout Washington you will make wonderfully weird discoveries. While wandering Seattle's spread of dispensaries, you can stay at one of the many cannabis-friendly historical Airbnbs, like the Bacon Mansion in Seattle's Capitol Hill neighborhood. Head out into the Olympic Peninsula, and you'll have the chance to swing by hot springs; not one, but two drive-in movie theaters; the quirky Olympic Sculpture Park; and the charming, refreshing pit stop that is Finn River Cider.

OLYMPIC PENINSULA

SEATTLE

OLYMPIC

WASHI

LEGALIZED

Medical in 1998,
recreational in 2012

POSSESSION

Adults over the age of
21 can possess: one
ounce of cannabis flower,
seven grams of extracts,
and sixteen ounces
of edibles

HOME GROWS

Only medical patients
can grow their own.

DELIVERY

Not legal

CONSUMPTION

Smoking is allowed on
private property, out
of sight.

CITIES

Olympic Peninsula
Seattle

SEATTLE   OLYMPIC PENINSULA

NGTON

RAVEN GRASS

A PURIST CANNABIS CULTIVATOR USING CREATIVE ILLUSTRATIONS AND PACKAGING TO DISRUPT INDUSTRY STANDARDS.

Raven Grass understands that cannabis is beautiful. So beautiful and awe-inspiring that it deserves to shine in its purest state, free of chemicals or harmful toxins. They stand by the beauty of their flower so steadfastly that they share every single nutrient and pest control method they use on or around their plants, on their website.

They understand that each strain is unique in its effects and created "Types" and "Hues" that correlate more accurately to their experiential nature. Laughing Buddha and Maui Wowie strains are categorized in the Gold hue, for example, described as Type 1, high-THC strains that come on with a giggle and bring a warm, sunshine high. They also feature artful packaging illustrated by my friend and Raven Grass co-founder, creative director Nichole Graf.

Graf co-authored *Grow Your Own*, a book about understanding, cultivating, and enjoying cannabis, and has long inspired me with her boundless creativity and good intentions. She started this farm with David Stein and Micah Sherman in 2013, but I didn't meet her until 2018, when I sniffed my way through her bouquet-filled terpene installation at *Broccoli* magazine's In Bloom festival. Graf had coordinated gorgeous floral and plant arrangements to reflect different individual terpenes found in cannabis like linalool (stress reliever) and myrcene (pain reliever), and all of us guests got to craft our own essential oil mixes with her various scented vials. Much like the thoughtfulness that went into that experience, the clever wordsmithing and cool designs for each product are more imaginative than so much of the industry, which is generally still reliant on the limiting binary of indica and sativa. Seeing such creativity, transparency, and a desire to set an example of how businesses can be motivated by more than mere profit — gives me a great deal of hope for the positively disruptive destiny of legal cannabis.

ravengrass.com

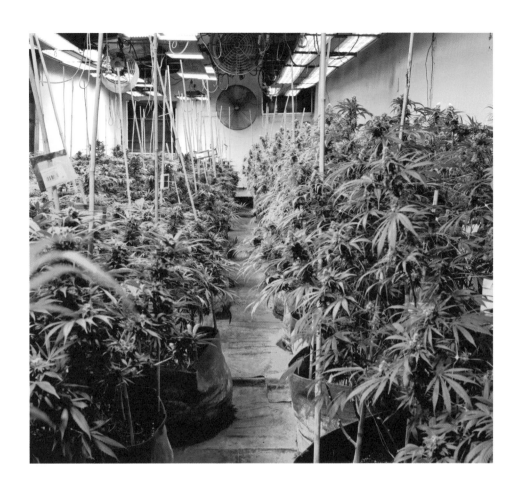

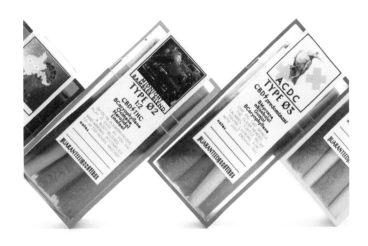

CHIMACUM CANNABIS COMPANY

A MUST-SHOP SPOT FOR FLOWER FIENDS LOCATED ON A PICTURESQUE FARM ON THE OLYMPIC PENINSULA.

There are many reasons to drive whatever distance necessary to partake in the joy of restocking at Chimacum Cannabis Company. *High Times* magazine and Washington growers alike consider it one of the best dispensaries in America, for one. For two, the farmhouse-styled dispensary is on a big plot of real, beautiful farmland with chickens roaming around. They also carefully source a flower menu that boasts nothing but craft-scale organic farmers, family-run indoor micro grows, and award-winning sungrown buds from interesting microclimates around the state. They offer all of this without a gram of pretension or weed snob energy.

Budtenders here are knowledgable and passionate about the plant, and they're happy to walk you through the weeds of terpenes, cannabinoids, concentrate varieties, and any other cannabis-related queries on your mind.

On the flip side, if you don't have any questions or don't know what you want and you just want to find some very good, fresh, pesticide-free, and less common strains, you're also in the right place. Chimacum is where my colleagues go for primo, small-batch buds from sought-after farms like Blue Roots, Raven Grass, and Eagle Trees—a bad-ass, sibling-owned operation out of Bellingham—plus award-winning CO_2 vapes from Doctor & Crook labs, delicious ginger-peach gummies from Verdelux Lush, and pink lemonade Pioneer Square bites.

Open Daily

9034 Beaver Valley Road
Chimacum, WA 98325

chimacumcannabis.com

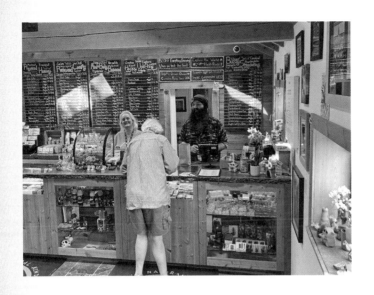

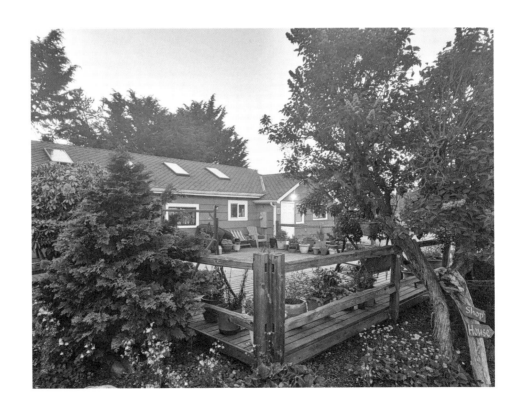

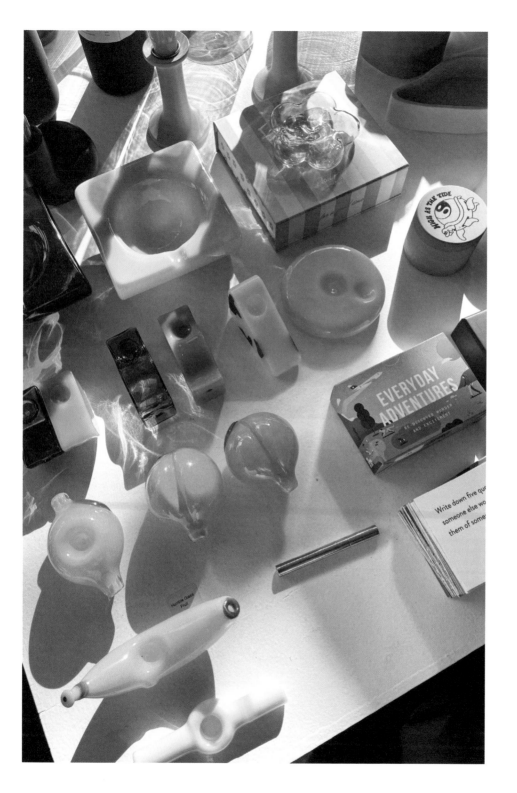

PRISM

A COOL INDIE BOUTIQUE OFFERING A RANGE OF UNIQUE CANNABIS-RELATED ACCOUTREMENTS.

I am a sucker for a cute space filled with handmade goods and interesting products from local artists and brands I've never heard of—the kind of place where you find a ceramic mug and knit socks for Mother's Day, an indulgent spa goodie for your friend going through a breakup, and a whimsically shaped candle or two for backup gifts. Prism is one of the Pacific Northwest's best versions of these eclectic shops, and one that's been cannabis-friendly since before it was socially accepted in the mainstream. It was also one of *Broccoli* magazine's first stockists when they launched in 2018!

You won't find cannabis at Prism, but you will be drawn in by their great selection of cannabis-friendly reads, well-vetted CBD skincare from makers like Herbivore, jade-colored glass pipes and bongs by Yew Yew, chic lighters too stunning to let anyone borrow, and imported Japanese incense to camouflage your sesh in the Airbnb later.

Open Daily

**5208 Ballard Avenue NW
Seattle, WA 98107**

prismseattle.com

HEYLO

A SEATTLE-BASED PROCESSOR RENOWNED STATEWIDE FOR ITS PREMIUM EXTRACTS AND TRANSPARENT LAB TOURS.

The world of cannabis concentrates is confusing to even the most experienced cannabis journalists due to its complex, scientific processing methods and the ever-expanding range of extract types, textures, and nicknames (there are a lot). Heylo is a processor that aims to alleviate some confusion by pulling back the cannabis industry curtain through transparency in their products, tours, and seasonal events.

Guests can have an inside scoop on how they process their high-quality, full-bud, pesticide-free plant material via CO_2 machines, taking every effort to keep the extract as close to the plant as possible for their strain-specific vape cartridges, topicals, and Heylo Jam—a saucy cannabis extract ready to dab or swirl on top of flower. With a background in chemistry and medicine, founder Lo Friesen came into this industry focused on the science. The more she learned about this plant, the more she realized how chemistry was at the center of it all.

"Chemistry is what determines how strains turn out and how they impact our bodies," Friesen explained. "I became determined to make this information as accessible as possible to the average person and to make extracts shine."

During Heylo's tours of their SoDo area facility—which happen every Tuesday and Thursday—the public is able to see every step of the cannabis extraction process. Visitors also get to take turns holding a ten-pound bag of weed, which tends to be exciting. They also regularly host Heylo Sessions, which are community events focused on bringing art, music, community, and cannabis education together. Whether through a yoga class in their lab or a party cruise around Lake Washington on a decommissioned ferry boat, the folks at Heylo aim to create space for people to feel inspired to do and learn something when they're high and connect with people they maybe wouldn't normally cross paths with. A true celebration of the way cannabis connects people in unexpected ways.

145 S Horton Street, Unit 1
Seattle, WA 98134

To book a tour, visit
heylocannabis.com

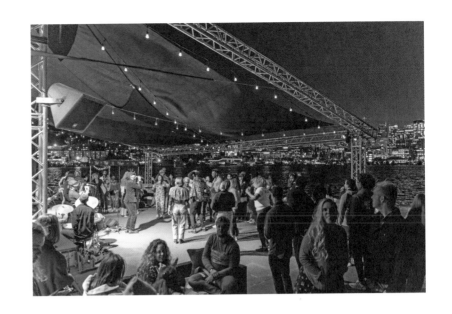

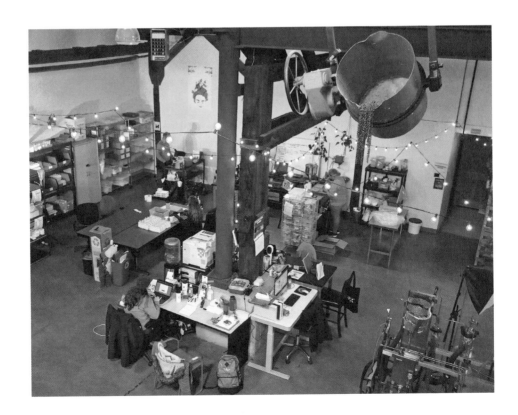

DOCKSIDE DISPENSARY & CANNABIS MUSEUM

A LONGTIME LOCAL FAVORITE WITH A COLLECTION OF ANTIQUE CANNABIS PARAPHERNALIA.

Dockside is a well-established local brand founded by three medical marijuana advocates who are dedicated to providing customers with a comfortable, well-stocked, science-forward shopping experience. Their location south of downtown Seattle in the "SoDo" neighborhood fits the bill perfectly. One corner of the space displays the Wirtshafter Collection of prohibition-era cannabis apothecary items, like vintage bottles of cannabis extract and remnants of century-old hemp products.

This brief Cannabis Museum is cool for obvious reasons, but what I love is how it provides historical context in a modern setting. Legally shopping for cannabis is a radically new experience for all of us today, but Americans have consumed cannabis for medicinal purposes long before it was

made illegal in the first place. Seeing the aged cannabis labels next to gleaming cases of pristine new products connects the dots in a powerful way. Founders Aaron Varney, Maria Moses, and Oscar Velasco-Schmitz reflect this medicinal legacy on another level by continuing to advocate for policy reform, like expungement of past criminal charges and the freedom to grow cannabis at home without permits, years after Washington went legal.

Open Daily

**1728 4th Avenue S
Seattle, WA 98134**

**For more locations, visit
docksidecannabis.com**

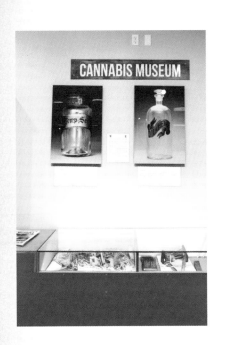

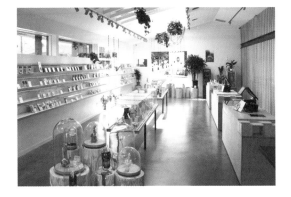

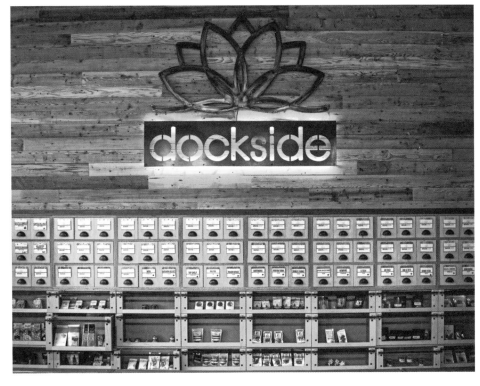

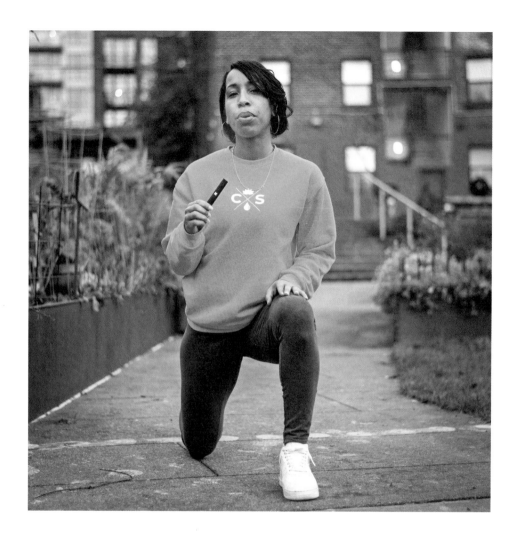

CANNASWET

CANNABIS CONSUMPTION-FRIENDLY WORKOUT CLASSES THAT MAKE SPACE FOR FOLKS WHO LOVE TO SMOKE AND SWEAT.

Felicia Tyson has led fitness classes for many years, but the first time she hosted one that included cannabis consumption, she found it totally changed the vibe of the class and the attitude of the attendees. More profoundly, it allowed Tyson to be her whole self while doing what she loves. Attendees had a blast, and it inspired Tyson to do more to help break down the stigma around cannabis and continue to find ways to combine cannabis and active lifestyles.

That first class in 2018 was more of a smoke-and-stretch sesh than her current-day CANNASWET boot camps at various public parks around the Seattle Metro, including Seward Park, three hundred acres of gorgeous Lake Washington views and ample space for respectful herbal consumption out of the way of fellow nature enjoyers. However, that *plein air* situation did not allow for year-round classes in the rainy Pacific Northwest, so in 2022, CANNASWET started partnering with licensed cannabis businesses with extra space on site, like Bellevue Cannabis, which has a fitness studio in its office.

In addition to yoga and mobility classes, Tyson has started offering the boot camp events of her dreams: serious HIIT workouts for people who love breaking a sweat while stoned. While each of the weekly and monthly classes are a little different, every class starts with a meet-and-greet with fellow classgoers and whichever farm reps are providing flower and vapes that day.

For class schedule, visit cannaswet.com

HASHTAG

A WELL-STOCKED, WHOLESOME SHOP KNOWN FOR ITS COMMUNITY-ORIENTED VIBE.

I mention this spot not just because they carry seemingly every Washington millennial's favorite gummies, Pioneer Squares (the brand behind all of my friends' favorite gluten-free, vegan edibles), but because of their relationship with their community, both in and outside of cannabis. A sweet, straightforward dispensary that's operated since 2015, Hashtag has a chill, no-frills vibe that never feels too fancy or too casual. The budtenders know their stuff, the space is filled with bright natural light, and it's great to bring your friends and family for a visit.

If you're starting your cannabis journey here, there's a range of playful pipes and iridescent grinders to choose from. But if you're a longtime consumer with a sky-high THC tolerance, they carry Journeyman's 100 mg Lemonade drinks, delicious and trusted vape cartridges from Heylo (see p. 92), or healing 1:1 CBD/THC tinctures from Fairwinds, a women-owned brand informed by ancient holistic concepts.

Since opening, co-founders Jerina Pillert and Logan Bowers have spent time advocating and testifying at the local and state levels for social justice reform. In store, they routinely accept clothing and food donations for Mary's Place, a nonprofit organization supporting women and families experiencing homelessness, and they've also sponsored a few pro-choice events in the region. Some might say, "What does weed have to do with abortion? Why get involved?" But the reality is legal cannabis is inherently political. These businesses are allowed to operate because of *legal* changes that unfairly haven't accounted for the people still serving time for or being burdened with a cannabis charge. It's our responsibility as industry professionals to keep advocating for legislative progress that prioritizes the health and well-being of the individual in all areas of social justice. I love to see dispensaries like Hashtag walking the walk.

Open Daily

**224 Nickerson Street
Seattle, WA 98109**

**For more locations, visit
seattlehashtag.com**

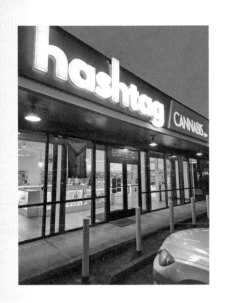

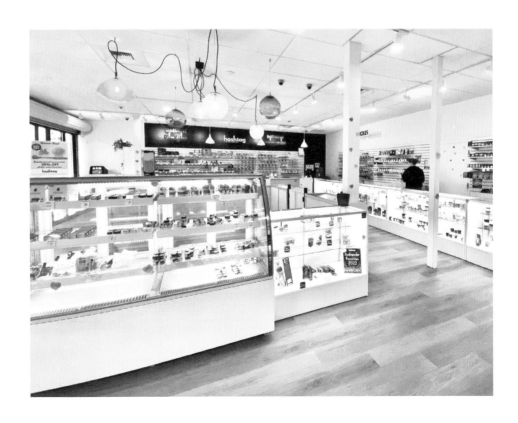

CANNA WEST

A RELIABLE FAVORITE WITH DEEP ROOTS IN THE CITY'S MEDICINAL SCENE.

Another shop that came highly recommended by my closest PNW confidantes due to its reliable, quality selection and community engagement, Canna West is the A+ version of a quaint neighborhood dispensary. Owned by Maryam Mirnateghi, longtime medical cannabis advocate and founding member of Washington State's Cannabis Ethics and Standards Board, this welcoming shop lives within a lovely Craftsman house with a modern retail space complete with a grand, tiled checkout area, big glass display cases, and digital menus on the walls. Despite the clean feel, Canna West boasts a warm ambiance with its honeycomb-inspired murals and knowledgeable budtenders who are experienced with talking customers through potency, dosage, and effects. As such, this is a great stop to bring more pointed questions about product recommendations for specific concerns, be it a good edible or tincture to help with falling and staying asleep or the right THC and CBD ratio in a topical to soothe carpal tunnel symptoms, for example.

Mirnateghi also owns the Canna West Culture Shop, a sister lifestyle store located directly across the street selling clothing, hemp CBD products, chic cannabis storage solutions, and vintage smoking accessories.

Open Daily

5440 California Avenue SW Seattle, WA 98136

cannawestseattle.com

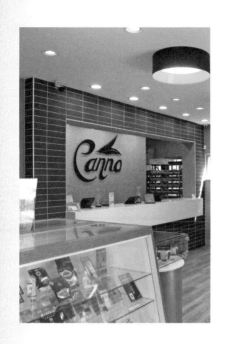

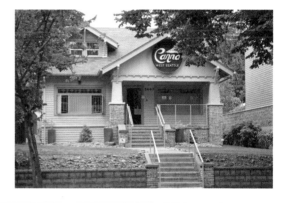

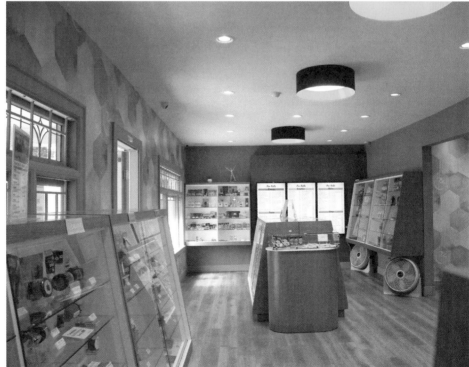

MOUNTAIN VIEWS TREE HOUSE JOINT

A GROUP OF WEED-FRIENDLY TREEHOUSES AVAILABLE TO RENT AND CUSTOM BUILT WITH NATURAL MATERIALS FOR A TRUE FOREST ESCAPE.

I believe that most everyone who appreciates cannabis also shares an appreciation for the imaginative and the weird. I'd go even further to say that most cannabis lovers are intrigued by experiences that feel special, experiences that transport you. Even if the Mountain Views Tree House Joint didn't happily permit the consumption of cannabis, I would consider this maze of architecturally inventive houses a truly magical destination for anyone with an affinity for the natural world. The four-acre property is filled with artistically built structures that are developed and crafted into nature with love by architect Tracy Rice.

Since 2013, she's added eclectically constructed tiny houses, lounge areas, and four fully functioning treehouses to the property—two of which, the Pot Leaf and Trippy, were built by legendary natural materials architect SunRay Kelly. These rentals are extremely tiny, with real walls and floors, a full bathroom, in-unit heat, and comfy bedding. Smoking accessories are provided, including a state-of-the-art Stundenglass gravity bong upon request, and guests are allowed to smoke cannabis inside and outside their lodging. It's glamping with a dose of Tolkien's Middle-earth and the scent of cannabis, all located less than an hour drive from Seattle.

As you can imagine, Rice is no average bud 'n' breakfast proprietor, offering ghost tours around Halloween and art workshops depending on the season and weather as add-on experiences. You might find yourself happy enough just wandering these mystical woods, gathering firewood for the communal camp fire, and stopping to pet the dogs, goats, horse, and pig that also call the Tree House Joint home.

mountainviewsbb.com

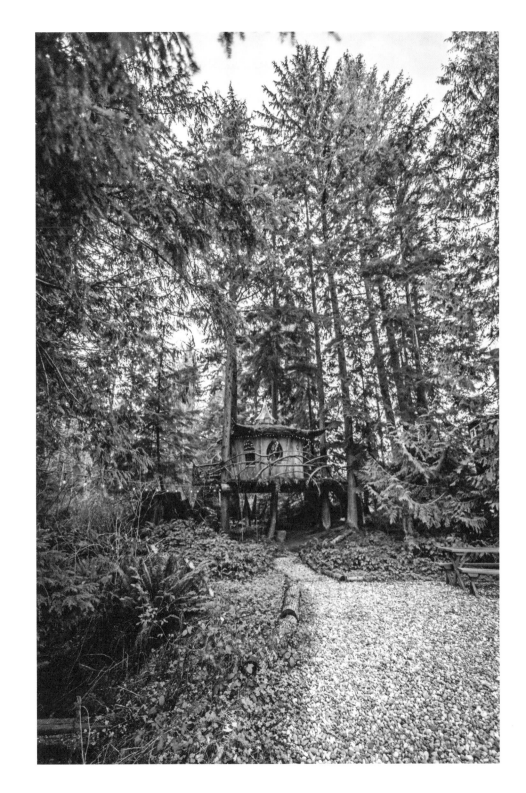

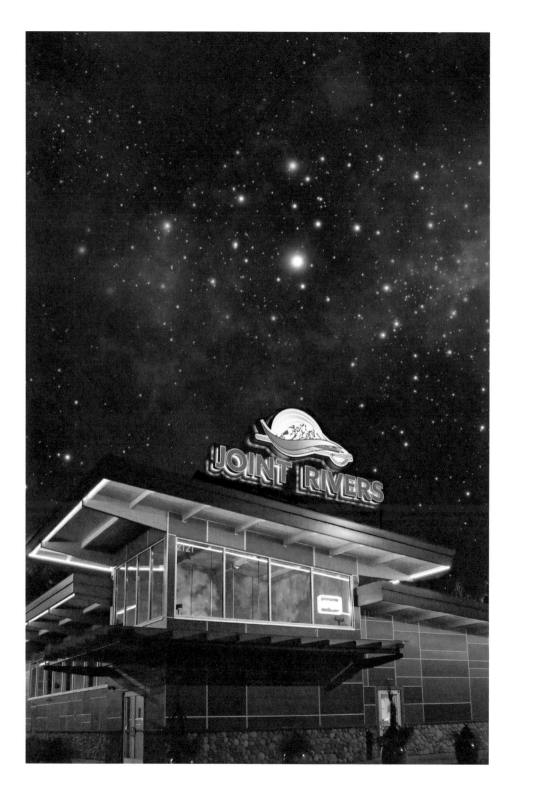

JOINT RIVERS

A LIVELY, CASINO-INSPIRED NATIVE-OWNED DISPENSARY OPERATING ON WASHINGTON'S MUCKLESHOOT TRIBAL LANDS.

In a smaller city called Auburn located just east of Tacoma, WA, lies the only cannabis dispensary in the state with drive-through service. This is because it's illegal to sell cannabis via drive-through in Washington's adult-use system. However, Joint Rivers is operated by the Muckleshoot Tribe, and, as a sovereign nation, they can essentially create and regulate their own cannabis programs on reservation land. The Muckleshoot Tribe is composed of descendants of the Native people who inhabited the Duwamish and Upper Puyallup watersheds of central Puget Sound for thousands of years before non-Native settlement, and, today, they're at the forefront of Washington's cannabis industry.

Although separate from the state's system, they still work with the state to a degree to stock state-licensed products, including familiar Washington goodies like Honu's infused peanut butter cups and Fairwinds' balanced 1:1 CBD/THC vape cartridges. Although it's very convenient to use the drive-through, if you've got the time, it's well worth parking to check out Joint Rivers' mid-century-styled building. They thoughtfully referenced the look of tribal casinos with the exterior design, lighting up the roof with bright neon color blocks that glow like beacons in the night. Inside, the clean, warmly lit interior reveals a well-organized selection of flower buds, pre-rolls, edibles, concentrates, vapes, topicals, and a fun selection of accessories including artful bongs. Although you won't find any slot machines here, the thrill of chance does find its way into the dispensary from time to time, but usually in the form of folks from the Muckleshoot Bingo Hall next door coming by to celebrate a win.

Open Daily

2121 Auburn Way S
Auburn, WA 98002

jointrivers.com

Montana's medical scene is long established, but the recreational scene has only just gotten underway. Since we're still within the first couple of years of legal cannabis sales in Big Sky Country, many cannabis professionals are idling in the "wait and see" zone (for now). There aren't many weed-friendly activities kicking off just yet, and most of the dispensaries in operation are respectable medical shops that have made the switch to cater to adult-use customers as well. That said, the cultivation of quality cannabis in Montana goes way back. There's an iconic bit of local lore regarding the Kurth family of Fort Benton, who, in 1985, tried out growing cannabis to save their failing cattle ranch. It worked so well that when they got to a point that they no longer needed to continue the risky business of illegal weed, the drug traffickers they had been doing business with did not accept their notice of resignation. The dealers pretended to be DEA agents and faked a raid, stealing the plants and reporting the ranchers to the real DEA afterward (nuts, right?).

To experience the most interesting parts of this nascent legal scene, I recommend heading outside of the bigger towns and over to Bozeman, where you'll find a more unique cannabis community emerging that includes my favorite titanium steel bong maker, Dangle Supply, the founder of which highly recommends picking up a kolache from Roly Poly Coffee Co. for a munchie pit stop before adventuring off into the unparalleled natural beauty with some freshly acquired greens.

BOZEMAN   WHITEFISH   BOZEMAN   WHITEFISH   B

MON

LEGALIZED

Medical in 2004, recreational in 2021

POSSESSION

Adults over the age of 21 can possess: one ounce of cannabis or the THC equivalent in other forms (eight hundred milligrams of edibles or eight grams of concentrate)

HOME GROWS

Adults may grow up to two mature plants and two seedlings at a time.

DELIVERY

Not yet, but medical shops have long been allowed to, so that's likely soon to change.

CONSUMPTION

Private property only

CITIES

Bozeman
Whitefish

WHITEFISH   BOZEMAN   WHITEFISH   BOZEMAN

TANA

JUNIPER CANNABIS

A BRIGHT BOUTIQUE DISPENSARY WITH OVER THIRTY STRAINS OF GREAT HOUSE-GROWN FLOWER.

Visiting Bozeman is about getting outside, getting dirty, and fully immersing yourself in Mother Nature's grandeur. Nestled in the Rocky Mountains, it sits just an hour north of the entrance to Yellowstone National Park. However, when it comes to restocking herbal supplies, even the most rugged adventurers will seek out the clean, serene interiors of Juniper Cannabis. Founders Adam Ryder and Jackie Worden—both lifelong cannabis and outdoors enthusiasts—wanted to create an approachable, boutique space that puts people from any walk of life at ease, utilizing natural light and wooden beams and floors to keep the neutral space feeling warm and inviting.

Ryder, born and raised in Bozeman, spent his youth poring over *High Times* magazines, fascinated by new methods of cultivation and eager to grow his own plants. He advanced in the medical market, and the shop's menu actually contains a few varieties that he's cultivated since the old days, like Montana Silver Tip, Blue Dream, and Unicorn Poop. All of the flower in store is grown at their advanced indoor growing facility, which sits on the Gallatin River. While known for their varied and consistently high-quality flower selection, you can experience the house strains in multiple forms, from dabbable concentrates to infused strawberry gummies and chocolate. You can also shop one of the coolest cannabis accessory brands around: Dangle Supply, a Bozeman-based maker of unbreakable titanium bongs and various other well-made, adventure-ready tools.

Open Daily

**120 N Grand Avenue
Bozeman, MT 59715**

**For more locations, visit
junipercannabis.com**

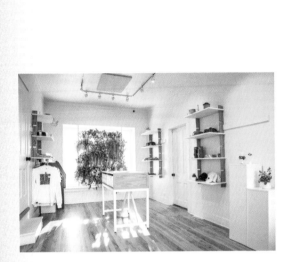

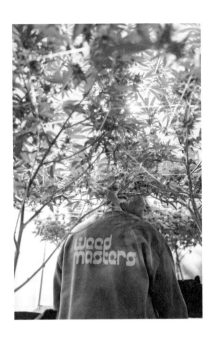

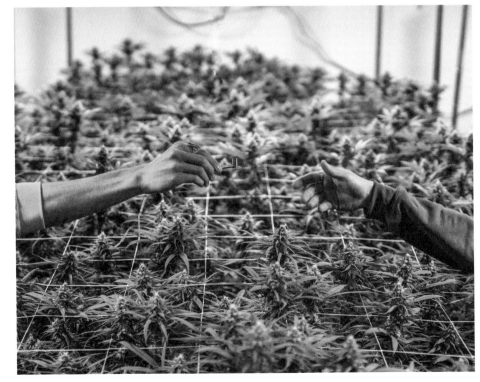

HASKILL CREEK FARMS

A MULTIFACETED HERBAL DESTINATION FEATURING A CANNABIS DISPENSARY, SPICE MARKET, AND WELLNESS BOUTIQUE.

If you find yourself in a small, naturally stunning town called Whitefish on your way to Glacier National Park, you can't not stop by Haskill Creek Farms, whether you're looking to restock on cannabis or not. This is the kind of multipurpose pickup destination that makes me very jealous of more flexible rules around cannabis retail in other states. Alongside homegrown flower, concentrates, and tinctures made from solventless hash rosin, you'll find a sprawling selection of medicinal herbs, spices and oils and an entire apothecary of botanical-based skin care.

Haskill Creek Farms is the kind of place that has something for every kind of Montana local and tourist. The founders call it a "modern wellness mercantile," and locals consider it

one of the best places to kick back and enjoy a panoramic view of the Flathead Valley and surrounding Rocky Mountains. All visitors to the store tend to be pleasantly surprised by the range of offerings, whether they came in for a ginseng supplement, Salt + Stone natural deodorant, organic olive oil, or a fresh eighth of cannabis flower. The menu is thoughtfully curated all around, and the shop itself is a beautiful, immersive farmhouse setting that feels like a special part of the surrounding community.

Open Daily

1202 Voerman Road
Whitefish, MT 59937

haskillcreekfarms.com

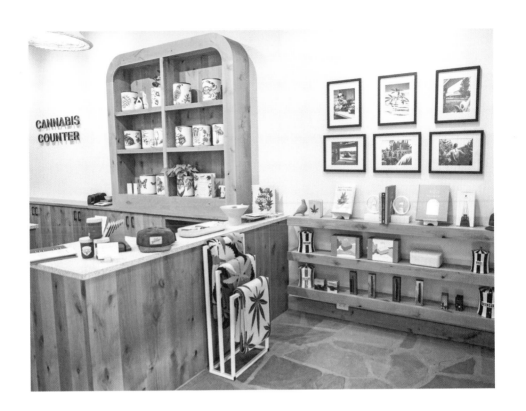

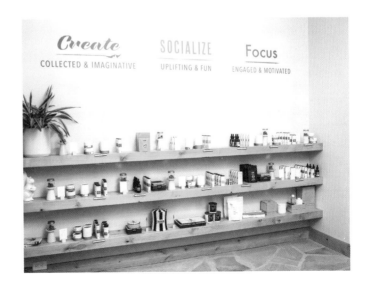

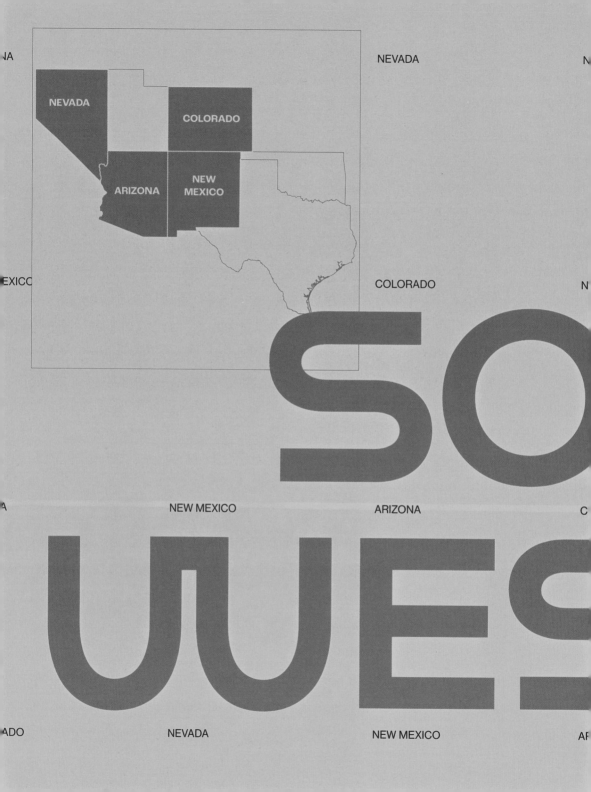

ARIZONA COLORADO NEVADA

THE

NEW MEXICO ARIZONA COLORA

UTH-

NEVADA NEW MEXICO ARIZONA

ST

COLORADO NEVADA NEW MEX

Arizona took its sweet time to legalize cannabis, but it learned from the states that came before it. Adult-use dispensaries opened their doors a matter of months after the voters submitted their ballots, including one of the only shops with a drive-through in the country. The community of cannabis farms and shops is still modestly sized, allowing them to foster a more united front against larger, multistate monopoly interests. Initial cannabis laws included social equity licenses, grants for small businesses, and consumption lounge elements—all things that other states have had to dedicate a lot of money and time to get amended years after legalizations. The cannabis scene brewing here is one being built to last and one you'll soon find out is worth adding to the must-experience list.

   Once you've consumed the best of Arizona cannabis, there is a piping hot food scene and the literal Grand Canyon to take in. Hype Phoenix restaurant Bacanora is on the to-eat list of gourmands everywhere, and Tucson's intoxicating mashup of cultures has fostered a vibrant haven for independent artists. If you head out to see natural destinations like Antelope Canyon, Camelback Mountain, or the floatable Salt River, just remember to bring more water and sunscreen than you think you need. To put it in the words of one dispensary owner I spoke with: "Don't be the person that requires helicopter rescue."

PHOENIX   TUCSON   PHOENIX

ARIZ

LEGALIZED

Medical in 2010, recreational in 2020

POSSESSION

Adults over the age of 21 can possess: one ounce of cannabis and up to five grams of cannabis concentrate or concentrate in edible form

HOME GROWS

Adults can grow up to six plants at home.

DELIVERY

Not legal

CONSUMPTION

Smoking is allowed on private property or in licensed consumption spaces.

CITIES

Phoenix
Tucson

TUCSON

PHOENIX

TUCSON

ONA

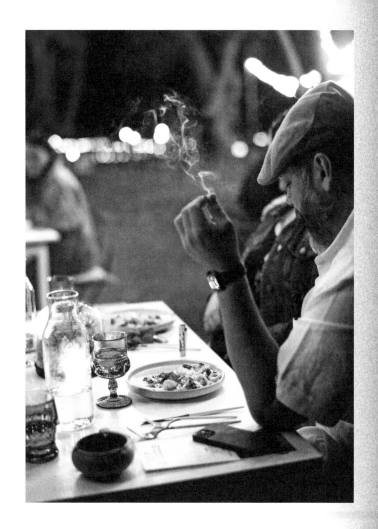

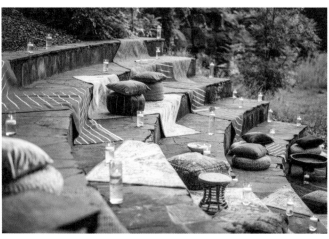

CLOTH & FLAME

IMMERSIVE, ONE-OF-A-KIND CANNABIS DINNERS HOSTED IN UNIQUE DESTINATIONS.

Cloth & Flame launched as a pop-up sensory dinner in the desert and since has grown into a prolific experience-design agency, producing hundreds of events per year in some of the most scenic outdoor destinations and iconic historic buildings in the US. They recently held a dinner in a Moab cave with David Blaine performing magic, and in the past they have flown tables into the base of the Grand Canyon. As founders Matt Cooley and Olivia Laux put it: "We create temporary venues and culinary experiences wherever they can be imagined." The company also pays property owners and parks passive income to ensure that the spaces they partner with remain unchanged and beautiful for generations to come.

Across all the experiences they craft, the cannabis dinners—their Verde Series—exude the utmost creativity. While the top chefs on staff get playful with terpenes as aperitifs, guests partake in entertainment like aura photography, an infinite mirror installation, stargazing through ultra-powerful telescopes, and a vibey hammock lounge between courses. Kicking things off with fast-acting tinctures allows guests to get on the same vibration then choose their journey from there. Guests have the option to turn on or off dosed elements at any time throughout the evening to tailor their experience to their cannabis comfort level. To encourage chefs to get adventurous with the infinite possibilities of combining cannabis and fine dining, the Cloth & Flame duo bring in plant chemistry experts for every event to lend scientific precision to the chef's ideas, ensuring each dinner is unique and enjoyable.

When I first chatted with Cooley for a feature in 2021, he said the Verde Series was influenced in part by a BBC show called *Mysteries of the Brain,* in which the host would play specific sounds and amplifications through headphones during bites of a meal, aiming to create intricate geographic sensations as people ate.

"I love the ability to create things that exist in one place at one time," Cooley said. And that's exactly what they've done here at Cloth & Flame.

For event schedule, visit clothandflame.com

GIVING TREE

AN INDEPENDENTLY-OWNED, MINIMALIST-CHIC DISPENSARY DESIGNED TO PUT NEWCOMERS AT EASE.

Lilach Mazor Power is a force in Phoenix's cannabis scene, juggling the Giving Tree dispensary, multiple cannabis product lines, and community and advocacy work as the vice president of the Arizona Dispensaries Association. Originally from Israel, Power moved to Arizona in 2006 and was inspired to enter the cannabis game when Arizona passed medical cannabis legislation in 2010. Her interest was, in part, due to her familiarity with the plant in her home country, where chemist Raphael Mechoulam first isolated THC, CBD, and the endocannabinoid system in the 1960s.

Once she was well convinced of her role in the cannabis industry, Power dove in, building out a modern, clean dispensary decorated with cascading houseplants. Her cannabis products include medicinal-leaning capsules and topicals under the name Kindred Cannabis and easy, breezy pre-rolls that go by Sneakers and Revelry. All of these products are made from plants grown, harvested, and processed in the north Phoenix community.

Open Daily

**701 W Union Hills Drive
Phoenix, AZ 85027**

givingtreedispensary.com

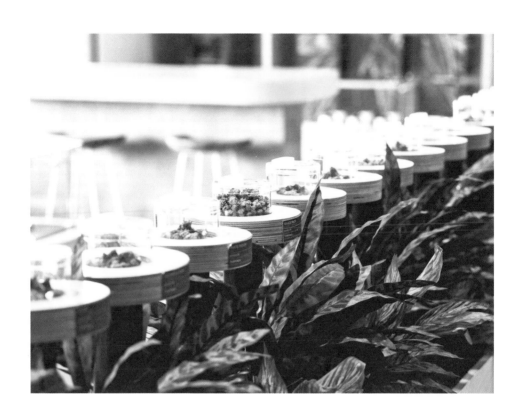

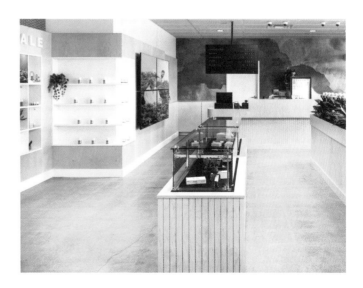

THE CLARENDON HOTEL AND SPA

A 21+ RETRO HOTEL WITH A LUXURIOUS POOL AND A FLOOR OF WEED-FRIENDLY ROOMS.

Within this boutique hotel lies a sixteen-room wing in which cannabis consumption of all forms is allowed. This is a big deal, as I can count on one hand the number of nicer hotels I could find offering consumption-friendly lodging. Originally opened in 1972, the Clarendon got a new owner in the early 2010s that embarked on a full renovation. They stayed true to the aesthetics and color palettes of the '60s and '70s with vibrant pops of lime green, red, and bright orange, and guests can achieve their Don Draper fantasy by ashing their joint contemplatively as they imagine prepping for their next business pitch.

You can't smoke outside of your room unless you're in the hotel's designated consumption lounge, but there's a retro pool area with a jacuzzi and a vibey rooftop space with lights and ample seating once you're adequately dosed and ready for fun.

The on-site Lazy Bee Spa is a full-service space offering luxurious facials, massages, body treatments, and waxing and the choice to add CBD topicals to any massage. Plus, there's also the Fuego Bistro restaurant serving tasty Latin fare. It's important to note that this is a hotel with cannabis-friendly floors, but it is not a weed-themed hotel. There are people who come here just to stay and not smoke, so be respectful. Still, this is an enormous step forward for true normalization of cannabis in public spaces.

401 West Clarendon Avenue
Phoenix, AZ 85013

goclarendon.com

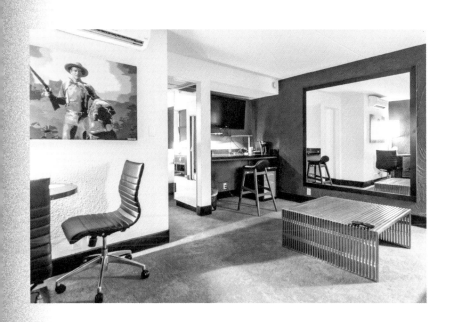

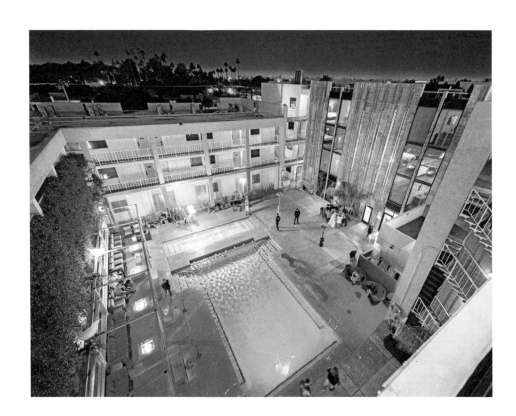

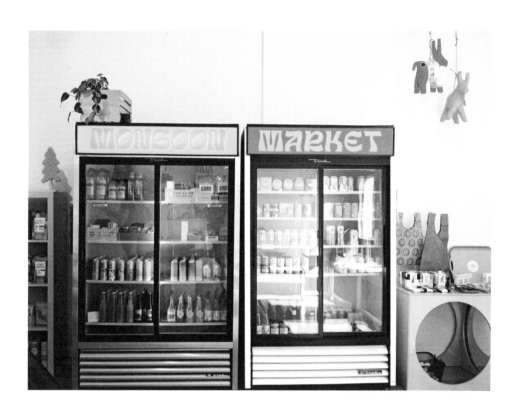

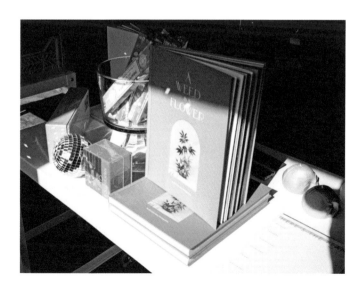

MONSOON MARKET

A CANNABIS-FRIENDLY WINE AND SNACK SHOP SELLING SMOKING ACCESSORIES AND HOSTING THE OCCASIONAL POT PARTY.

Think of the coolest neighborhood wine shop you've ever seen, then add in interesting snacks, home goods, and a living room in the middle of the shop, and you're in the ballpark of Monsoon Market. First on my radar as a stockist of *Broccoli*'s gorgeous puzzles and Yew Yew's chic glass pipes, this shop specializes in natural wine and stocks a ton of non-alcoholic beverages, exclusive pantry items, vintage homeware, and fun gifts, from Baggu bags to sweet, squiggly candles. Flower children can also find the iconic Hamburger Grinder from Another Room

(yes, a smooth-grinding weed grinder that looks like an adorable burger) and organic, psychedelic-patterned rolling papers made with food-safe dyes from Field Trip. If you enjoy cannabis, cute things, and good treats, this wine shop is the ultimate Phoenix-area pitstop for munchie supplies.

Open Daily

**3508 N 7th Street, Suite 140
Phoenix, AZ 85281**

monsoonmrkt.com

SUNDAY GOODS

A CANNABIS BRAND WITH MODERN DISPENSARIES BRINGING NEW ENERGY TO PHOENIX-AREA NEIGHBORHOODS.

This cannabis brand led the charge of stylish cannabis in the Southwest. I recall admiring their chic, midnight-toned packaging from afar, mentally noting that there was something intriguing germinating in this part of the country. Sunday Goods' vertically integrated operation offers whole flower buds and pre-rolls grown at their sustainability-minded indoor facilities, as well as oil cartridges extracted from that flower—all consistently delicious and aesthetically pleasing among the other essentials in one's purse.

Both stores—Phoenix and Tempe—are quite honestly stunning, with creative design that utilizes clean lines and interesting tile and wood elements to elevate the space. The 5,000-square-foot Tempe location offers complimentary kombucha and cold brew while you shop—one reason I truly envy Tempe residents. Sunday Goods doesn't just deliver on refreshments (although I love a sophisticated, thirst-quenching atmosphere as much as anyone else); they also prioritize efficiency. Yes, I'm talking about the drive-through. This is one service that very few (potentially zero) state governments are OK with, and one we typically don't associate with higher-end experiences. But if you could get fine dining via a drive through, wouldn't you try it out? On a rushed afternoon, when I have other errands to run before heading home, hell yes I would!

Open Daily

**723 N Scottsdale Road
Tempe, AZ 85281**

**For more locations, visit
sundaygoods.com**

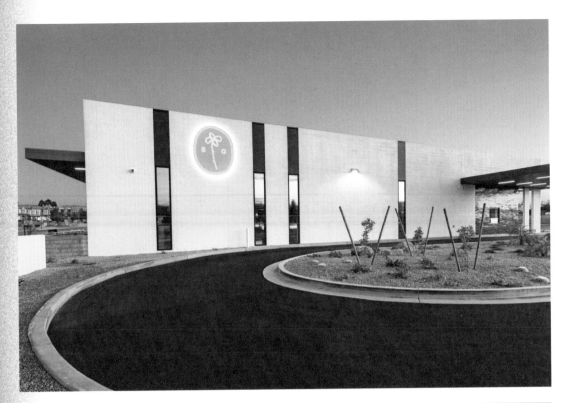

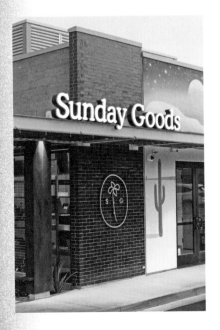

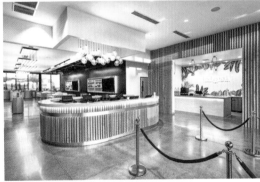

BOTANICA

A STYLISH, LOCALLY OWNED DISPENSARY DESIGNED TO HONOR THE NATURAL DESERT BEAUTY OF ITS HOME STATE.

Co-owners Jennifer Slothower and Bryan Hill met in the marching band while attending the University of Arizona, perhaps partook in some desert greenery together, and the rest was history. They've worked together, became certified sommeliers together, and, for the past decade, carved a path in cannabis together. When bringing their dream dispensary to life, the pair wanted to celebrate the aesthetics and energy of Tucson and the Sonoran desert, so they embraced the idea of a desert mirage to create a shady, dream-like sanctuary working with designers to bring the concept to life.

The optical illusions that make us see a shimmering mirage in the distance are referenced with reeded glass elements—that wavy-looking textured glass—and thoughtful elements of light and shadow, depending on the time of day. As sommeliers, they aim to correlate the typical wine-tasting experience with cannabis, adding an emphasis on consumer education with every product recommendation.

"Everything on the menu is something that every member of our staff has personally tried and can stand behind, from the fellow family-owned Canamo Concentrates to CBD tea and beverages by Waveland," Slothower said.

Open Daily

6205 N Travel Center Drive
Tucson, AZ 85741

botanica.us

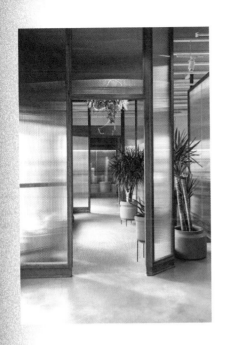

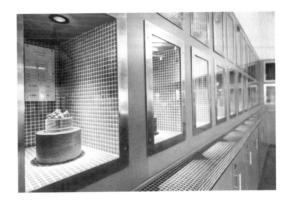

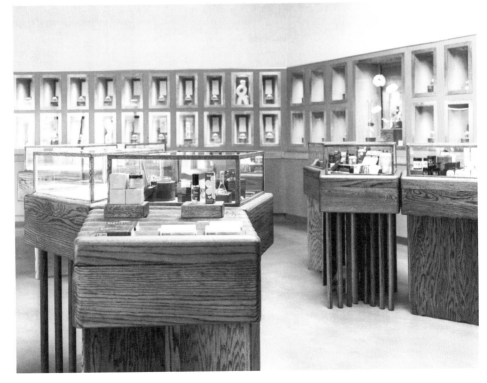

After over ten years of legal cannabis business in the state, a new chapter of Colorado cannabis is emerging. Many popular shops and experiences have come and gone—RIP to the sushi-and-joint-rolling workshop—and many out-of-staters formerly making regular re-up visits no longer have to cross any borders to access legal pot. The glory days of being the first state to legalize may have faded as the majority of states pass their own medical and adult-use laws, but now that the kief dust has settled, it's allowed for the seeds of the second wave of businesses and experiences to take root. It also revealed the parts of Colorado cannabis culture that will stand the test of any amount of time or global pandemic, from the psychedelic murals and daily laser light shows within the International Church of Cannabis to Jad's Mile High Smoke lounge, which is essentially a cannabis sports bar without the beer.

Although known for its dynamic landscape of high desert, plunging river canyons, snowy Rocky Mountain peaks, and ancient ancestral Puebloan cliff dwellings in Mesa Verde National Park, Denver proper carries plenty of its own treasures to behold. Head through the right faux bookshelf and you'll find yourself in Williams & Graham, a true speakeasy-style bar. And if you spot a giant milk container in the distance, that isn't the edible you ate earlier; it's Little Man Ice Cream, a hype dessert destination for the whole family. If Aspen's more your speed, keep reading to find the high-end cannabis offering to match any luxe ski resort getaway.

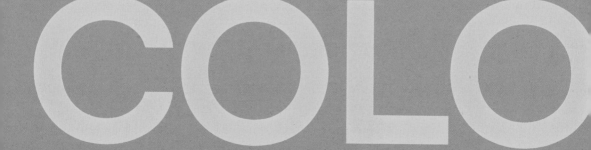

VER   ASPEN   DENVER   ASPEN

COLO

LEGALIZED

Medical in 2000, recreational in 2012

POSSESSION

Adults over the age of 21 can possess: one ounce of cannabis flower, eight grams of concentrates, and eight hundred mg of THC in edible form

HOME GROWS

Adults can grow up to six plants and three flowering plants at one time.

DELIVERY

Yes, but only to private residences (no hotels).

CONSUMPTION

Smoking is allowed on private property and licensed consumption lounges.

CITIES

Denver
Aspen

DENVER

ASPEN

DENVER

RADO

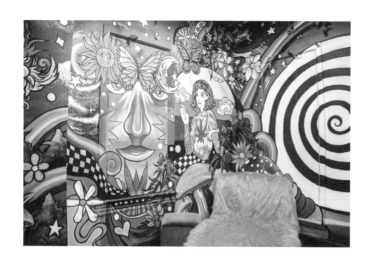

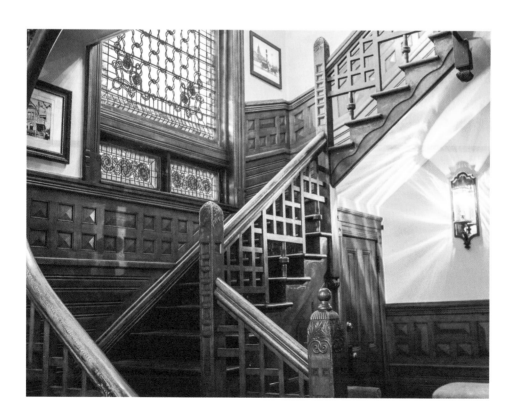

MARIJUANA MANSION

A MANSION STEEPED IN CANNABIS HISTORY CONVERTED INTO A MULTI-ROOM MUSEUM.

Of all the chapters of this 135-year-old sandstone mansion's existence, I imagine that being Marijauna Mansion is the most fun it's ever had. Originally built in 1889 by esteemed Denver architect John J. Huddart, this is now a charming, one-of-a-kind spot where history and weed are celebrated with black light posters and period-appropriate furnishings. I appreciate how autonomous this experience is: walk-ins, selfies, and self-guided tours are all welcome. Guests can also use the space as a studio for cannabis-friendly photoshoots and private rentals. There's something incredibly refreshing about the lack of pretension and judgment at a place listed on the National Register of Historic Properties.

Rooms in this mansion have been remodeled and custom-decorated with cannabis-centric themes, many selfie-ready punctuations of neon lighting, and comfortable, sumptuously furnished seating for impromptu smoking seshes and/or photoshoots.

The coolest thing is the legit cannabis history related to this building: It earned the nickname "The Marijuana Mansion" in 2012 when it was the Colorado headquarters for the Marijuana Policy Project (MPP). At the time, the mansion was also home to the offices of the Vicente Sederberg law firm, which worked with the MPP on Colorado's cannabis legislation. This is where the world's first successful recreational cannabis bill (Amendment 64) was written to legalize cannabis in Colorado.

Open Thursday–Sunday

**1244 Grant Street
Denver, CO 80203**

mjmansion.com

LOVA CANNA CO.

A TRUSTED LOCAL CHAIN OF SHOPS LOCATED IN DESTINATION NEIGHBORHOODS ACROSS DENVER.

This growing group of shops started with the Edgewater location just outside of Denver, where the first legal sale of cannabis happened right when Colorado's market kicked off. Power couple Amanda Fox and Matt Shifrin have developed this brand with care to maintain the neighborhood shop vibe with each outpost, ensuring all locations are stocked with house flower, slick disposable vape pens, and delectable berry gummies.

The stores have a uniform sophistication, with clean, simple interiors and open floor plans, and there's a pleasant ease here that reflects the mix of clientele. There's no pressure to interact if you'd like to browse on your own time, and the budtenders are well-versed on cannabis science and ready for any questions from an industry insider or a first-time toker.

Overall, LOVA Canna Co. is a good place to go for interesting brands you've likely heard of and always wanted to try, like ioVia tinctures, low-dose 1906 edibles and flower, and uber-potent Rick Simpson Oil from the highly reputed Green Dot Labs. One aspect I personally love about LOVA shops is that they're here for the night owls; most of their locations are open until the legal cutoff: 11:45 p.m.

Open Daily

3121 E Colfax Avenue
Denver, CO 80206

For more locations, visit
lovaco.com

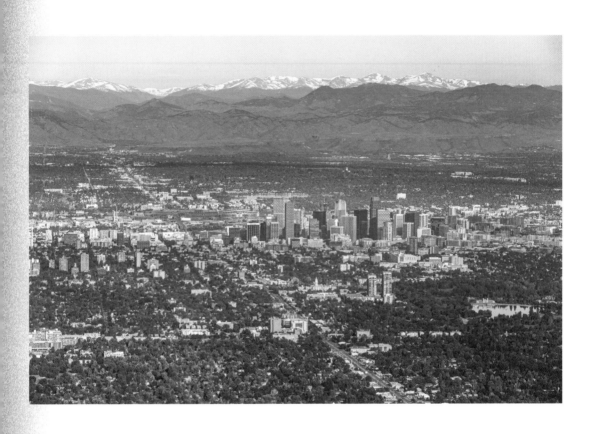

WANDA JAMES, CO-FOUNDER OF SIMPLY PURE DISPENSARY

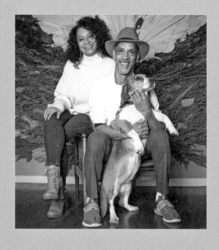

As the first Black owners of a legal cannabis store, a cultivation facility, and an edible company in America, Wanda James and her husband, Scott Durrah, are both pioneering entrepreneurs and celebrities in the cannabis industry. As a couple experienced in both grassroots politics and restaurant management, they were the best possible business partners to assume this major responsibility.

In those early years, James spoke thoughtfully to many major media outlets about bringing equity to the cannabis system at large, focusing mostly on the issue of cannabis-related arrests continuing to disproportionately impact Black and Brown people and the need for immediate expungement assistance. This level of community activism as well as their ability to balance the needs of cannabis consumers, newcomers, and regulators seriously contributed to the wave of cannabis legalization that followed.

These days, James juggles CEO duties at Simply Pure, ongoing advocacy work, and regent responsibilities at the University of Colorado with family life at home with Durrah, an acclaimed cannabis chef, and their three dogs. I caught up with James over the phone to chat about the Denver scene and her dreams for American weed.

WHAT DO YOU LOVE ABOUT DENVER'S CANNABIS SCENE?

A lot of people use the word "oversaturated," which I resent. We're just mature; this is what it looks like. I think Denver is a phenomenal place for cannabis, with many dispensaries that offer different experiences, just like a healthy restaurant scene. It's a controversial thing to say, but I also think Denver is the true Napa Valley of cannabis. Yes, there are rich roots of cannabis legacy in Northern California, but Denver as a city is where cannabis is being celebrated as a whole, and the climate is just as kind to fantastic cultivation.

HOW HAS SIMPLY PURE EVOLVED SINCE IT FIRST OPENED ITS DOORS IN 2010?

These days, any week of any month, there are incredible cannabis chefs hosting dinners, including my husband and Chef Harold Sims (@haroldforhigher on Instagram), who won an episode of Netflix's *Cooked With Cannabis*. The city is evolving along with the cannabis scene; the neighborhood where our store is located was known as the North Side for a long time, but if you ask someone who's moved here recently, it's "LoHi." It used to be a predominantly Latino, working-class neighborhood, and it's transformed into a destination area with lots of hype restaurants, ice cream shops with a line around the block, and lots of cool Airbnbs.

WHAT WAS YOUR MINDSET WHEN DESIGNING YOUR STORE?

Our space was designed by Kim Miles, who's now the host of *High Design*, a dispensary makeover show on Discovery+. I wanted it to be a beautiful space that could help destigmatize cannabis while staying true to our roots. It needed to feel safe and warm; we were intentionally going for Whole Foods rather than an Apple store. When you first walk in, there's a fourteen-foot floral display made out of dried flora that's all native to Colorado. Then, you're welcomed by "budologists" who are trained for two months prior to hitting the sales floor. Some people come here for relief from back pain; others stop by to consult on a cannabis flower boutonniere they're planning for a wedding.

WHAT ARE SOME LOCAL BRANDS YOU RECOMMEND?

1906's edibles are one of our favorites. Very modern company making low-dose edibles that use beneficial herbs to support each edible's goal, i.e. active, focus, etc. Coda Signature Truffles [offers] artful, hand-painted chocolates by a Paris-trained chocolatier. Our Simply Pure CBD dog treats are great, too, but I'm biased.

WHAT ARE YOUR HOPES FOR THE CANNABIS SCENE IN GENERAL?

In many ways I love watching what's happening; in lots of ways we're failing miserably. We haven't done a good job of looking out for small businesses. I'm sad we're continuing to operate in this legally illegal space that limits small businesses from thriving. Because we can't access federally insured banks, we still spend $50K a year just to have a bank account. I would love to be able to tour a farm and sample flower like you can at a winery, but we can't do that. I would love to attend a wedding on a beautiful farm, but we can't do that. America is built on small business, not corporate giants. There are ongoing limitations that are killing the creativity of what cannabis could be.

COLORADO CANNABIS TOURS

A LONG-ESTABLISHED HOST OF WEEKLY CANNABIS TOURS, PUFF-AND-PAINT CLASSES, AND TONS MORE.

Don't let their modest name fool you—this company is one of the most active figures in Colorado cannabis tourism. Their signature Colorado Cannabis Tour brings guests to a state-of-the-art cannabis cultivation facility and two dispensaries via a cushy party bus. They also offer limo options, a concentrate tour, a brewery and dispensary tour, and a ton of experiences across the city every week, from Introductory Cooking with Cannabis, where you learn how to make your own infusions, to private cooking classes for you and a few friends. Depending on the status of their partnerships with local spots, Colorado Cannabis Tours also hosts cannabis-friendly karaoke nights. Their most popular offering

is probably their weekly Puff, Pass & Paint experiences, which provide paints, brushes, canvases, and any other required art supplies and invite attendees to bring whatever form of cannabis they'd like to consume.

These accessible, inclusive classes are less about honing one's painting techniques and more about getting stoned and painting at whatever skill level while making unexpected friends with the range of folks who find themselves in one of these classes. Sometimes, that's exactly what the day calls for.

For class registration, visit coloradocannabistours.com

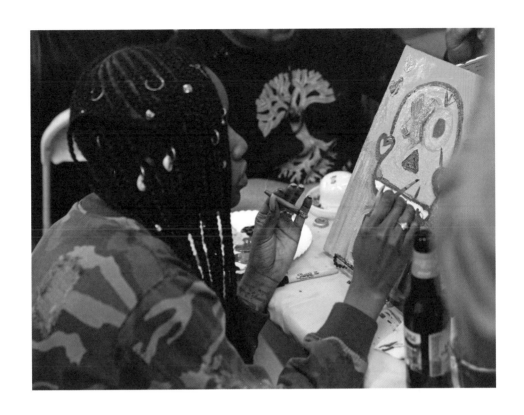

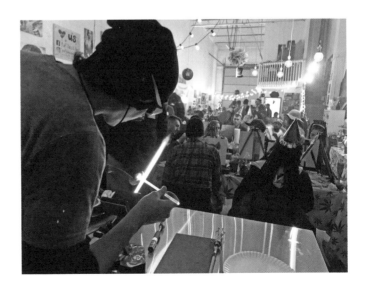

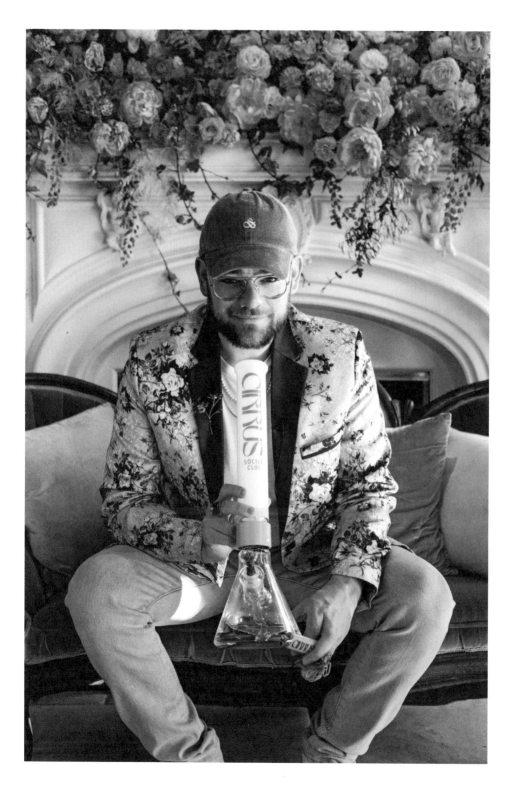

CIRRUS SOCIAL CLUB

A FIRST-CLASS CONSUMPTION LOUNGE WHERE GUESTS CAN ENJOY PREMIUM DABS BENEATH CHANDELIERS.

Although Colorado was the first state to legalize cannabis, it wasn't until 2021 that Denver revamped its local regulations to allow for home delivery services and "hospitality establishments," i.e. public consumption lounges. When that happened, hospitality and cannabis media veteran Arend Richard knew it was time to create his dream cannabis experience. In 2018, the Denver native founded the cannabis media platform WeedTube and, in 2020, co-hosted the Glitter Bong Bash, the first major cannabis event for the LGBTQ+ community.

"I say Cirrus is like nothing that's come before, not because people are consuming cannabis here, but because we went all-in on the luxurious environment unlike anywhere else in cannabis," Richard explained, noting their custom coral Steinway & Sons piano and the giant crystal chandeliers overhead.

"We want to be the adult Casa Bonita— the spot that people have to see when they're in Denver."

While I can attest that Casa Bonita remains a surreal, memorable experience that anyone who appreciates the strange should see at some point, unlike Casa Bonita, I anticipate visiting Cirrus Social Lounge a second, third, and likely fourth time.

3200 E Colfax Avenue
Denver, CO 80206

cirrussocialclub.com

LEIFFA

POSSIBLY THE MOST TRUSTED CULTIVATOR, PROCESSOR, AND DISPENSARY PACKAGE IN DENVER.

Great flower comes down to cultivators and the seeds or clone from which it grows. But processors understand great flower in their own way, as they're the ones extracting dabbable, vapable concentrates from plant material, and if they want to create high-value concentrates, it requires an understanding of quality plants. I think one of the reasons Leiffa came so highly recommended from my friends in Denver is because co-founders Brandon Epley and Eryc Klein started out as processors, and it shows in the quality of every flower, oil, and edible product on their shelves.

When these childhood friends came together in Denver in the mid 2010s with the goal of getting into the cartridge game, they soon learned about solventless extraction processes and totally changed their direction. Using a relatively simple combination of ice, water, heat, and pressure was an appealing alternative to constructing a whole extraction laboratory for butane or CO_2 extraction. However, it also meant zero room for flaws

in the plant material. Whatever you spray on those plants, you're going to taste, so growing their own flower was their safest bet to ensure they produced consistent, quality flower for extraction. Since they had a processing facility making rosin, it didn't take much effort to start making strain-specific gummies for targeted effects.

Now that rosin is the concentrate form du jour, they're at the forefront of the Denver/Lakewood scene and a desirable destination for live rosin cartridges. The houseplants and welcoming neon signage set a cheery tone as soon as you walk into the lobby of the store, which leads to an open, streamlined bud room of products, merch, and well-curated glass smoking accessories.

Open Daily

**6900 W Colfax Avenue
Lakewood, CO 80214**

leiffa.com

PATTERSON INN

CANNABIS-FRIENDLY LODGING IN STUNNING HISTORIC SUITES, LOCATED IN THE CENTRAL CAPITOL HILL NEIGHBORHOOD.

The coolest thing about modern cannabis businesses operating in really old spaces is that at an earlier point in its lifetime, that building probably did host a smoke sesh or two. Patterson Inn's sandstone chateau was first built in 1891, so it's totally possible that the early occupant—congressman and publisher of the *Rocky Mountain News* until 1913, Thomas M. Patterson—sparked up some devil's lettuce with visiting writer friends prior to Prohibition. Today, the building is one of the few, proud cannabis-tolerant establishments on the National Register of Historic Places.

The Patterson Inn features nine rooms in a bed-and-breakfast atmosphere, with an on-site consumption lounge for guests to enjoy some local greenery. They don't sell product here—guests need to bring their own—but they do offer non-alcoholic refreshments and a food menu that can be customized to complement the flavors or effects of the cannabis you're consuming. There's also a tavern on the basement floor of the hotel, but I'm more excited about the made-to-order, complimentary breakfast that changes every day. A proper wake-and-bake is best paired with eggs and bacon in my book.

420 E 11th Avenue, Suite 12
Denver, CO 80203

pattersoninn.com

CHEF ROILTY

A MICHELIN-TRAINED CHEF WHO PUTS CANNABIS FIRST AT HIS PRIVATE DENVER-AREA DINNERS AND CLASSES.

When Jarod Farina left Florida for Colorado in 2011, he had no intentions of becoming a weed chef. He was busy processing cannabis into coveted concentrates and winning awards at early underground events like Los Angeles' Secret Cup. It was during that particular trip out west that he was offered a job at a processing lab in Colorado, and he planted roots down in Denver without a second thought. Over the next few years, he made a home in the city's cannabis community as the medical scene developed and voters legalized the plant for real.

It was in 2015 that he decided to apply his cannabis processing skills to more culinary purposes, infusing every snack for a New Year's Eve party, which was—surprise—an enormous hit. He started going by the name Chef Roilty, teaching cooking classes and training with chefs at major restaurants that include the Michelin-starred Joel Robuchon restaurant in Las Vegas. Farina has also made appearances on TV shows including *Beat Bobby Flay*, *Chopped 420*, and Bravo's *Southern Charm*.

These days, Farina offers private classes and next-level dinners that tourists routinely visit Denver to enjoy. Whether it's a two-top date night, an off-season meal for professional football players, or an annual 4/20 feast, Farina offers a cannabis-centric fine dining experience that goes beyond just gourmet edibles.

Take the Chef's Canna Leaf Pasta experience, for example, which serves fresh pasta dough that's been rolled into sheets, laminated with fresh cannabis fan leaves (the big ones, with the seven points), and cut into pasta. It's then served with an herby cream sauce with grated cannabis leaf on top and placed atop a perforated pillow that's been filled with cannabis smoke for a dramatic, hazy arrival to the table.

Clearly, Farina is a sucker for fanfare, and I love it. You can expect over-the-top sensory elements like dry ice for foggy drama and special smoke tools with almost every meal.

For event schedule, visit chefroilty.com

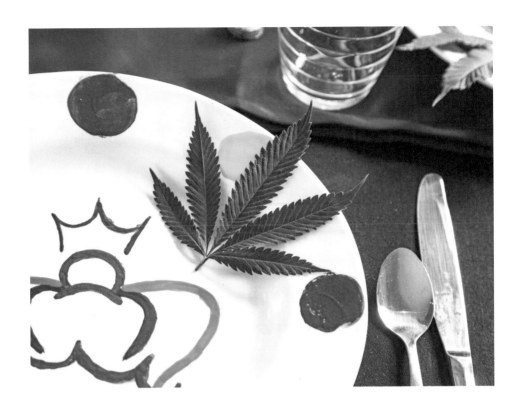

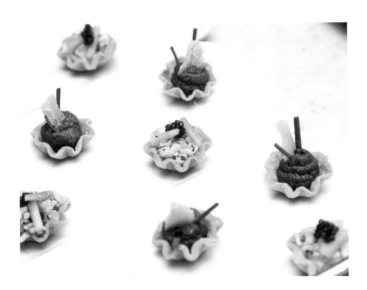

DALWHINNIE FARMS

A BOUGIE GIFT BOUTIQUE, CANNABIS DISPENSARY, AND FARM DESIGNED FOR ASPEN'S JETSETTERS.

Dalwhinnie Farms is not messing around. There's no being coy or beating around the bush here; the first thing you see when you enter the store is a seemingly life-size golden horse statue. This is a luxurious answer to the question "Where are all the upscale dispensaries that speak to the chic destinations of this outdoors-oriented state?" Located in a historical building that was renovated to feel like a jewelry store, Dalwhinnie Farms stocks premium house-grown flower alongside actual diamond jewelry and other fine goods. Dalwhinnie's actual cannabis farm is located on a 210-acre horse ranch at the base of the San Juan Mountains, where the flower is sustainably grown.

The beautiful, midnight blue jars of flower and cartons of joints offered here are hand-trimmed and hand-rolled, which is an increasingly rare find in these mature markets and an example of the substance behind the style at Dalwhinnie Farms. This family-owned company aimed for extravagance when opening, but they're very in tune with the older, truer ethos of the region: that enjoying nice things doesn't mean being a snob. This is a cool place to simply witness cannabis sold alongside show pieces like a $14,700 fully crystal saddle made by Aspen-based artist James Vilona, but it's also a great place to stock up on good flower when you find yourself in town for the Jazz Festival. You could also pop in to shop the Dalwhinnie Farms-branded cashmere blankets, apparel, gold ashtrays and grinders, or candles scented with their signature blend of champagne, black currant, and lily of the valley. Or you can feast your eyes upon the equestrian-inspired leather goods, cannabis leaf jewelry with real diamonds by Jacqui Aiche, Nomatiq all-crystal pipes from Brooklyn, and Badash crystal ashtrays.

Open Monday–Saturday

**108 S Mill Street
Aspen, CO 81611**

dalwhinnie.com

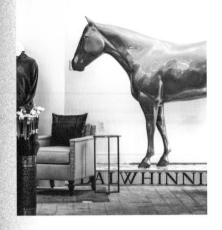

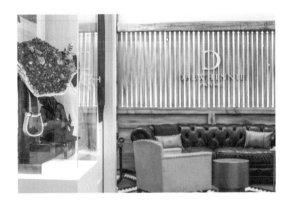

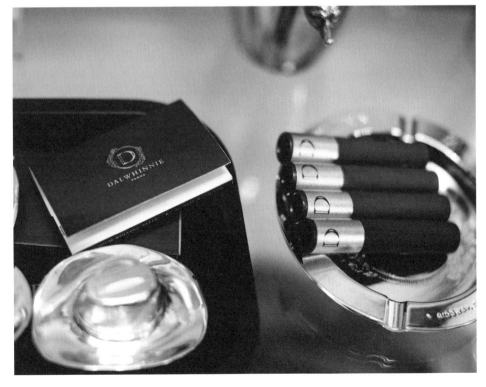

Let's be real: no one comes to Las Vegas for weed. This is a destination for raucous, flashy, high-risk fun, which isn't the type of vibe one typically associates with cannabis. That said, when I visited Las Vegas for my twenty-first birthday, I would have traveled far to get some fresh flower for morning-after recovery. Fortunately for any cannabis-minded visitors, times have changed, and legal cannabis is becoming a part of the Sin City experience more and more with each passing year. Legal dispensaries designed with the extravagant mindset of casinos, weed-centric weddings, and a weed-themed magician at one of the popular night clubs in town (Smokus Pocus) are just the tip of the iceberg. However, just because it's Vegas does not mean it's a weed-friendly free-for-all.

Since casinos are federally regulated, you absolutely cannot join tobacco smokers and light up inside casinos. On the flip side, shops can be open as late as they want here, and many are open 24/7. Laws change all the time, so it's possible that the next time you're in town, a licensed lounge will be operating out of the Cosmopolitan Hotel, but for now, keep your cannabis indulgence away from the hotels and casinos.

The best way to do Sin City's weed scene is to know where you're going, check in with your hotel or Airbnb about any special deals or partnerships with a particular shop in town, and expect that the multiple music festivals, business conferences, and bachelorette parties happening on any given weekend may seriously impact your wait times in-store.

LAS VEGAS   LAS VEGAS   LAS VEGAS   LAS VEGAS

NEV

LEGALIZED

Medical in 2000, recreational in 2017

POSSESSION

Adults over the age of 21 can possess: one ounce of cannabis flower, edibles, or topicals and 3.5 grams of concentrate

HOME GROWS

Residents can grow up to six plants at home, but only if they live more than twenty-five miles from a dispensary.

DELIVERY

Yes, but only to private residences (no hotels or casinos).

CONSUMPTION

Smoking is only allowed in private residences or licensed consumption spaces.

CITIES

Las Vegas, baby!

LAS VEGAS   LAS VEGAS   LAS VEGAS   LAS VEGAS

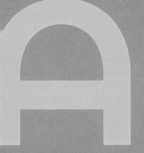

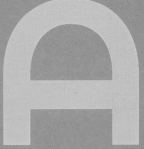

ADA

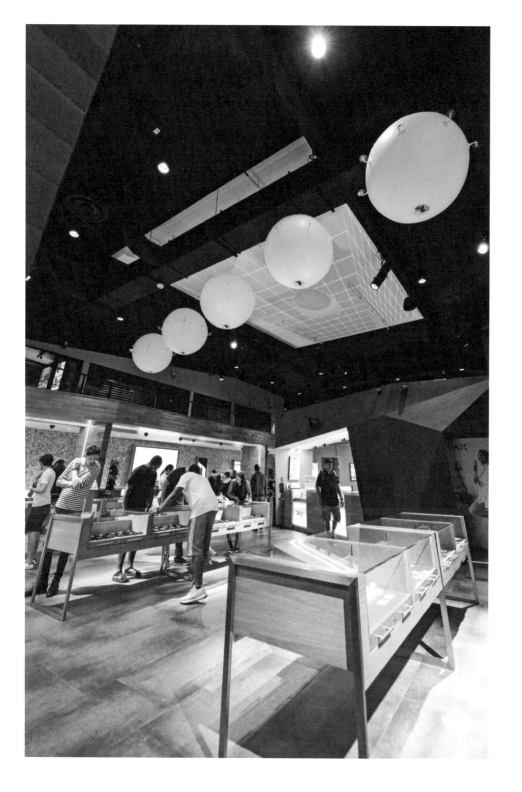

PLANET 13

AN EXTRAVAGANT, CASINO-INSPIRED DISPENSARY—THE LARGEST IN THE WORLD—LOCATED RIGHT OFF THE STRIP.

If you ask anyone about Las Vegas cannabis, "Planet 13" will likely be the first words to cross their lips. From fifteen-feet-tall metal lotus flowers illuminated with LEDs on the roof to the towering water feature out front and the manufacturing robots that put on "light saber duels" in their free time, this shop is so extra and *very* Vegas. You can even get married here in a cannabis-themed, state-recognized ceremony (Elvis impersonator is not included). Typically, I would not recommend a shop purely because of the extraness, but in Planet 13's case, the degree of over-the-top fanfare is so high altitude that I can't help but give the company props for leaning all the way in.

Because of its must-see aura and the challenge of getting around Las Vegas in a timely manner, many tourists make this spot their only pot stop during their trip. That means that product here moves fast and flower stays fresh. Even when I spoke with locals about their recommendations, they mentioned this "tourist trap" because, at the end of the day, the assortment is always well-stocked with interesting brands, big and small, and weekly fresh drops of flower, edibles, and concentrates. Moving that many people through their doors each day also means they've streamlined their pre-order/pick-up system to run without a hitch, and budtenders are well-accustomed to answer questions from customers across the spectrum of cannabis experience.

For out-of-towners, the space accommodates more than just cannabis needs; inside the same expansive building, there's a full-on greenhouse-inspired restaurant offering non-infused Mexican-American fare, artisan pizzas, twelve beers on tap, and craft cocktails. Of all the extra bells and whistles available at Planet 13, the free shuttle service to and from most hotels located along the Strip may be the clincher. You *don't* want to mess with Lyft's surge fees in this city.

Open 24/7

2548 W Desert Inn Road, Suite 100 Las Vegas, NV 89109

planet13lasvegas.com

NUWU NORTH CANNABIS MARKETPLACE

A PAIUTE TRIBE-OPERATED DISPENSARY WITH A VAST CONSUMPTION LOUNGE AND UNIQUE FLAVOR.

There is the Strip—the contemporary core of the Las Vegas experience—and then there's the historic heart of Sin City located a little to the north, aka The Fremont Street Experience. This is where, in 1906, the first Las Vegas Hotel was built and where the first neon-adorned high-rise broke ground in 1956. Although this stretch of Fremont has turned into its own sort of amusement park celebrating Las Vegas history, it retains a lot of the nostalgic charm of Old Vegas that you associate with Elvis movies and the like, offering a slightly more chill pace of partying.

NuWu Cannabis Marketplace is like the Fremont Street Experience of the other Las Vegas Strip shops. Operated by the Las Vegas Paiute Tribe, this is a long-established shop located near Fremont Street that operates within Tribal legislature, meaning they're able to do things other dispensaries can't, like have a 24/7 drive-through and a spacious, slick consumption lounge way before everyone else was permitted to get going.

In 2023, NuWu opened the doors to its two-story, 40,000-square feet dispensary, which includes a three-acre consumption-friendly courtyard and a Sky High Lounge with views of the Fremont Street Experience. If you're heading out to take in the crimson-hued natural beauty of Red Rock Canyon National Conservation Area, you can stop at NuWu North along the way. At either location, you can trust you'll find kind, well-versed budtenders and a solid selection of flower, edibles, and concentrates.

Open Daily

1235 Paiute Circle
Las Vegas, NV 89106

For more locations, visit
nuwu.vegas.

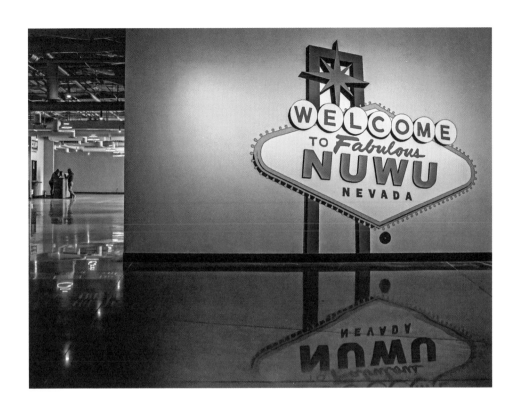

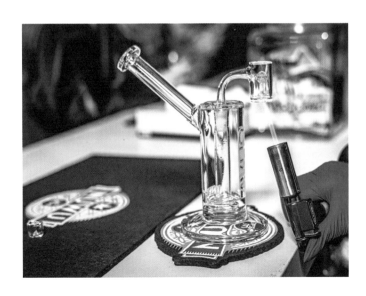

THE LEXI

LAS VEGAS'S FIRST 21+, CANNABIS-FRIENDLY HOTEL, COMPLETE WITH A POOL AND A SEXY, SOPHISTICATED VIBE.

One of the newest hotels in town is also the city's first official cannabis consumption-friendly hotel. Formerly the Artisan Hotel on West Sahara Avenue, a multimillion-dollar renovation transformed and elevated the grounds with totally refreshed lodging, including a lounge, chapel, pool, and a Cajun-inspired steakhouse overseen by Executive Chef Jordan Savell of *Hell's Kitchen*.

From the same team that developed the Clarendon Hotel in Phoenix, the Lexi follows a similar model, requiring all guests to be over the age of twenty-one and restricting cannabis consumption to one floor of the hotel (where very high-grade air filtration systems have been installed). Unlike the Clarendon, however, the Lexi has a definitively sexy vibe,

with high-drama design, rich splashes of black and scarlet from floor to ceiling in the lobby, and the option to sunbathe topless around the pool.

As city and state regulations evolve, the property intends to update where and how consumption can take place, but for now, no smoking is allowed around the pool area, no matter how vibey the shaded day-beds are. The playful, flirtatious hotel aims to normalize cannabis in travel and offer a new, slightly off-Strip venue for more intimate pool party events throughout the spring and summer.

1501 West Sahara Avenue
Las Vegas, NV 89102

thelexilasvegas.com

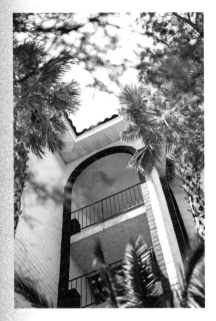

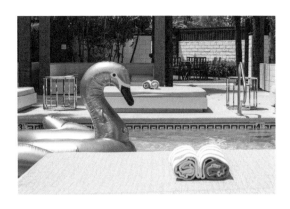

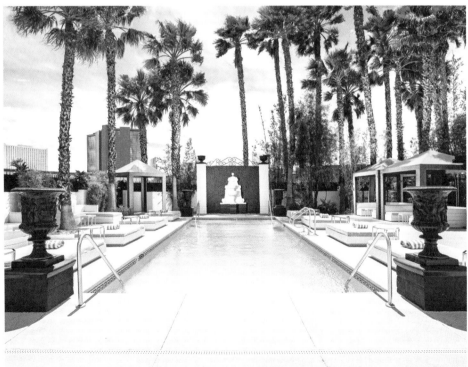

New Mexico's scene is one of the fastest to get on its feet—much to the excitement of many tourists visiting one of the wondrous natural destinations here. Hundreds of shops are in operation in the state, and many of them are selling above-average flower for affordable prices. The abundance of sun in this desert state makes outdoor cultivation a popular choice, and the plants seem to thrive in this soil. This climate may be arid, but after thousands of years of human civilization—from ancestral Puebloans and beyond—the land offers many regions of rich, unique terroir from which dozens of farms are proud to harvest.

While legal cannabis in New Mexico is new, its cannabis culture is not. There's a long-established hippie presence here, thanks to visits from icons like Aldoux Huxley and Bob Dylan seeking mind-expanding experiences and wide-open space for creative inspiration. The modern landscape has yet to reflect those psychedelic roots, though. Beyond the hundreds of dispensaries in operation, the legal space is still finding its groove (consumption-friendly lounges and activities have yet to really kick off). Fortunately, head a few miles in any direction and you've got broad vistas of natural beauty at your fingertips that many cross multiple state borders to enjoy. I cannot wait to see and sample more New Mexico-grown cannabis as this scene develops.

ALBUQUERQUE   SANTA FE   FARMINGTON   TAOS   ALBUQUE

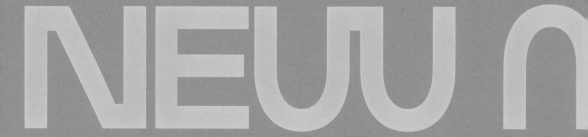

LEGALIZED

Medical in 2007, recreational in 2021

POSSESSION

Adults over the age of 21 can possess: two ounces of cannabis, sixteen grams of cannabis extract, and eight hundred milligrams of edible cannabis

HOME GROWS

Adults may grow up to six mature plants and six seedlings at a time.

DELIVERY

Yes, but only to private residences (no hotels).

CONSUMPTION

Smoking is allowed on private property or at a licensed cannabis consumption area.

CITIES

Albuquerque
Santa Fe
Farmington
Taos

SANTA FE   FARMINGTON   TAOS   ALBUQUERQUE   SANTA FE

MEXICO

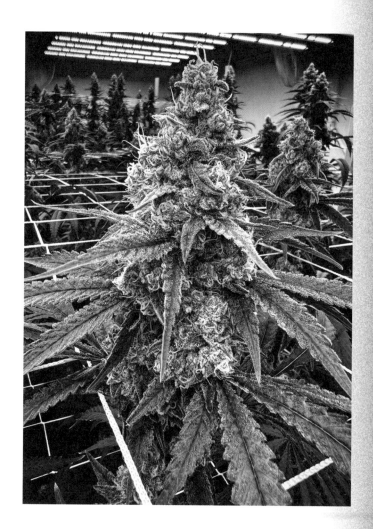

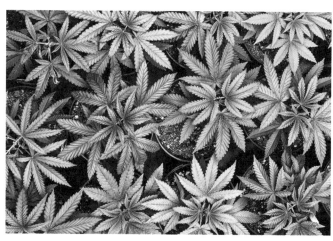

CARVER FAMILY FARMS

A CANNABIS DISPENSARY, CLONE NURSERY, AND PLANT AND CACTI BOUTIQUE OPERATED BY OLD FRIENDS.

As New Mexico's largest city, I assumed my research would turn up a broad range of unique spots to shop and experience; however, one name continued to come up: Carver Family Farms. A couple sentences into my conversation with co-founder Mathew Muñoz—a fifteenth-generation New Mexican—and I understood why.

It turns out that Muñoz's family has a land grant from a Spanish King that dates back centuries! Mind-blowing, right? The grower at Carver Family Farms is actually his old friend and co-founder, Andrew Brown, who he met while working at a headshop. Brown was the glass blower/resident flower dealer out back, and since they linked up, Muñoz hasn't smoked anyone else's flower. Erika Brown is the third co-founder and helps cultivate the high-quality, indoor-grown flower that Albuquerque residents seek out.

Their petite farmstand of a shop—a literal "microbusinesses"—only stocks house flower, and the concentrates and vapes are all made with house-processed live resin bubble hash. The team has always intended to maintain quality, not quantity, so you might have to make two trips in order to catch an eighth of their signature Carver strain, bred by Andrew in-house. That's no inconvenience when there's numerous other plants to peruse in-house. CFF also grows award-winning cacti and succulents as well as hard-to-find peppers like Dragon's Breath, Death Spiral, and heirloom aleppo chilis—all of which you can buy as living plants inside the dispensary.

Open Monday–Saturday

**8917 Adams Street
Albuquerque, NM 87113**

carverfamilyfarm.com

RISING ROOTS

A HORSE-FRIENDLY FARM SUSTAINABLY GROWING CANNABIS, VEGETABLES, AND MEDICINAL HERBS.

Lindsay McCoy was born and raised within miles of her cannabis farm, where she and her family have grown vegetables for years. Their smokable flower is grown in the sun alongside the rest of the farm's bounty, fed the same organic fertilizers and protected by the same ladybugs serving as pest control for the other greens grown on-site. McCoy also utilizes a highly efficient irrigation system that uses 60 percent less water than conventional methods, setting an admirable example for all Southwestern states growing cannabis in or near drought-ridden areas.

Perhaps one of my most favorite things about Rising Roots is that this farm *loves* the art of responsible cultivation—in every sense. Her sons have even developed a community farmstand, aptly named Little Roots, so all young cultivators in the community can sell the food they grow.

"One of the goals for the Little Roots farmstand is to get enough kids collaborating and growing together so that we can donate surplus food to the Rio Grande food bank to help beat the hunger crisis in New Mexico," McCoy explained.

She plans on partnering with other nonprofits that support small rural New Mexico communities as well as organizations providing cannabis education to parents, children, and families. Not only does this farm cultivate its own cannabis, but it also houses and cares for horses, which is such a precious visual. Three horses currently reside on the farm, and McCoy proudly sits on the board for the New Mexico Horse Rescue.

"It is very rewarding," she added. "Working with horses is a beautiful way to stay connected to your inner strengths and intuition."

risingrootsnm.com

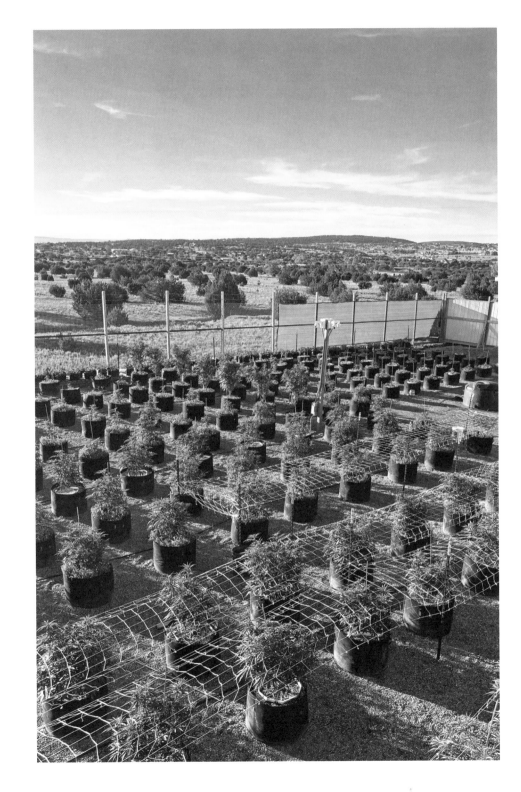

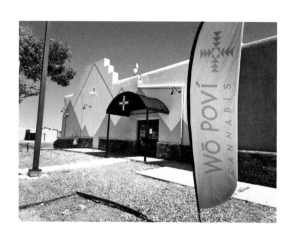

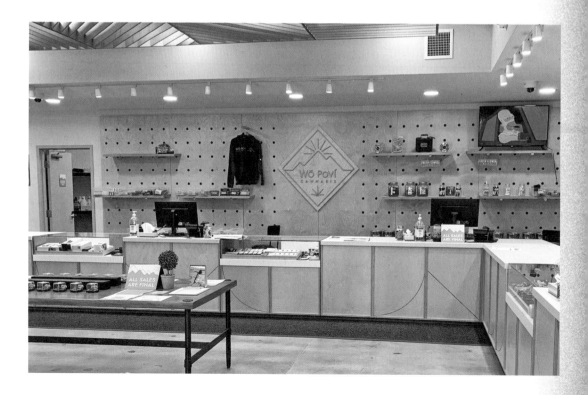

WŌ POVÍ CANNABIS

THE FIRST NATIVE-OWNED SHOP IN THE STATE— AND ONE OF ITS MOST THOUGHTFULLY OPERATED.

In the native Tewa language, *Wō Poví* translates to "medicine flower," which is a fitting name that also speaks to the deep Indigenous roots in this part of the state. Wō Poví Cannabis sits on the tribal lands of the Pueblo of Pojoaque, one of the smallest tribes in the state today, but it's also located in the homelands of the Ancestral Puebloans who are now spread out on reservations and sovereign land across the Four Corners region connecting New Mexico, Colorado, Arizona, and Utah. In fact, you can still see ancient cliff dwellings at the nearby Bandelier National Monument that date back to between 1150 and 1600 AD.

You get the best of the old and the new at Wō Poví, where familiar brands like Cheeba Chew edibles are sold alongside niche craft farms like Close Encounters Farms and Iron Fist Cannabis, but the difference here is that the tax revenue goes straight back to the Pueblo tribe. The shop—formerly a small casino—has been renovated to reference pueblo architecture and features a floor-to-ceiling mural of the verdant Pojoaque Valley inside. Lots of skylights give the interior an airy feel, while locally made art and historic photographs tell more of the story of the tribe as you browse. As much as the space is built with cannabis newcomers and tourists in mind, the clean, welcoming environment was just as vital in getting the tribal elders on board with a legal weed enterprise.

Open Daily

68 Cities of Gold Road
Santa Fe, NM 87506

wopovicannabis.com

LAVA LEAF ORGANICS

A FAMILY-OPERATED SANTA FE DISPENSARY STOCKED WITH A COLLECTIVE OF SUN-GROWING CULTIVATORS.

This collective led by New Mexico natives is focused on growing cannabis rich in terpenes and cannabinoids without the use of synthetic chemical pesticides or nutrients, and through a collaborative multi-grower farm model, changing the conversation around sustainable cultivation altogether.

"We have adopted the Japanese principle of *kaizen*—continual improvement of our systems, community, and community members," said Tony Martinez, CEO and co-founder of Lava Leaf Organics.

Tony, along with his brother Mitchell Martinez (resident plant whisperer) and their father Steve Martinez, go beyond strategic, efficient use of resources to actually leave the soil more healthy than when they found it.

"We are proud of the fact that we are improving the land below and around our pots and beds because the living soil's microbial colonies and earthworm populations grow and spread throughout the land, which helps the surrounding soil hold more water over time and supports a more diverse array of life forms far beyond the bounds of the grow," Martinez explained.

To make up the Lava Leaf Collective, the family works with fifteen different contractors and individuals who are all dedicated to cultivating with ever-improving methods. In the store, welded chain and heavy-duty steel furnishings pay homage to the hard-working blue-collar community they serve and are a part of. The space is modern and industrial, but grounded by soulful elements like a full "chakra-tuned" set of crystal singing bowls aimed to amplify their healing intentions. Martinez hopes to help all cannabis consumers access sustainably cultivated flower, but part of the family's healing intentions is to empower those consumers to continue this conversation in other cannabis spaces by asking questions like: How was this grown? Was water and power sustainably used? Does this company recycle? Are the growers or creators of this product valued by the owners of the farm? These are all questions I hope spread beyond New Mexico's borders and into the cannabis industry as a whole.

Open Monday–Saturday

**5100 E Main Street, Suite 105
Farmington, NM 87402**

lavaleaforganics.com

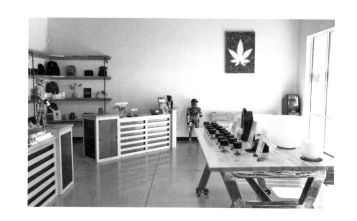

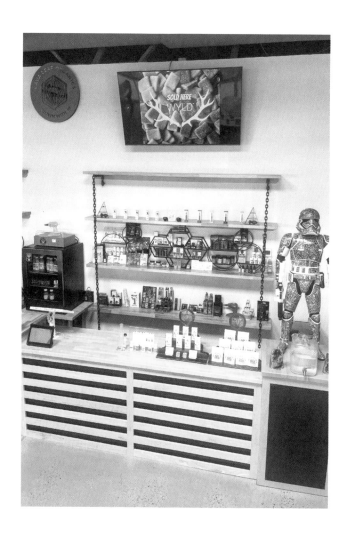

BIGHORN WEED CO.

A FAMILY-RUN, VETERAN-OWNED DISPENSARY OFFERING CRAFT FLOWER OUT OF A RENOVATED BLACKSMITH SHOP.

Ekin Balcıoğlu and Steve Weiner arrived in the 6,600-person town of Taos without really looking into it. They just wanted to be somewhere other than Los Angeles during the darkest point of the COVID-19 pandemic. They fell in love with this place in a matter of days, though, and they never left. It could've been the mystical sunsets or the powerful history pulsing through the city in the form of the Taos Pueblo, a UNESCO Heritage Site and Native American community that has been continuously inhabited for over one thousand years.

"People talk about the audible, sensory 'hum' of the desert here. It's real," said Weiner, who worked on a licensed cannabis farm in Humboldt before he'd ever heard of Taos, NM.

Once the state legalized cannabis, he saw an exciting opportunity to try things again in their new home, and perhaps help build a more successful environment for smaller, craft operators than California's brutally competitive market. While the couple set about renovating a historic building that formerly housed a blacksmith shop, they started getting to know farms and launched a delivery-only store—the only delivery option north of Santa Fe, in an area that currently doesn't even have pizza delivery.

"We believe you should know where your weed comes from and how it was grown," Weiner explained. "We handpick small batches of cannabis from licensed farms that consciously grow in tune with our planet."

Bighorn Weed Co.'s partners for grams and joint packs include Rising Roots, Taos Mountain Budz, and Gold Fish Farms—two of the three being New Mexican women-owned and operated. Inside the store, you'll find stunning original wood features revealed by the historic renovation, curated art on the walls, and gardening books and indie magazines on the shelves that lend a living room energy to the space, beckoning folks to hang out for a while. The magazine selection includes Weiner and Balcıoğlu's *Hamam Magazine*, a publication dedicated to bathing art and culture—perfect reading material for a stay at the legendary Ojo Caliente Mineral Springs Resort & Spa a couple towns over.

Open Tuesday–Sunday

536 Paseo Del Pueblo Norte
Taos, NM 87571

bighornweed.com

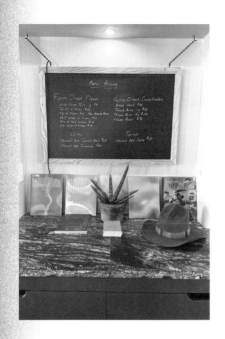

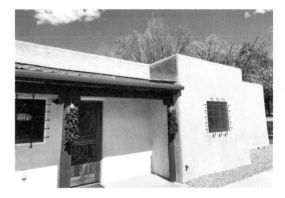

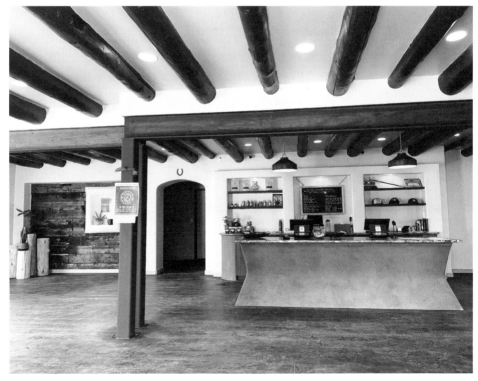

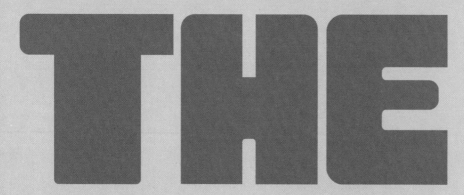

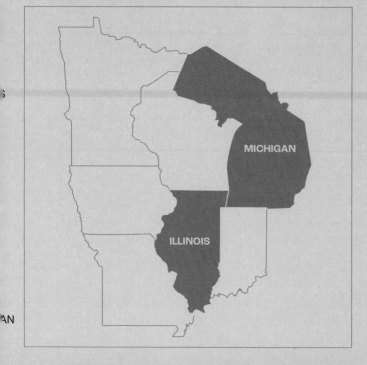

ILLINOIS   MICHIGAN   ILLINOIS

MICHIGAN   ILLINOIS   MICHIGA

MID·
VEST

ILLINOIS   MICHIGAN   ILLINOIS

MICHIGAN   ILLINOIS   MICHIGA

When Illinois legalized cannabis, they kind of changed the game. It was the first state to legalize recreational sales through an act of the state legislature, as opposed to voter initiatives. It was also the first to enact a comprehensive social equity program to attempt to build an industry with a more equal playing field from the ground up. Unfortunately, the residency requirements aimed to benefit economically disadvantaged locals and communities most impacted by disproportionate arrests during the War on Drugs resulted in a slurry of lawsuits from the moneyed folks impatient to access those coveted licenses. Nearly a year after legalization took effect, there wasn't a single licensed cannabis business statewide that was majority owned by a person of color. Instead, the existing owners of licensed medical cannabis businesses, who were allowed to immediately grow and sell in the recreational program, raked in the initial hundreds of millions in sales.

We're now entering the second wave of legal cannabis in Illinois. The lawsuits holding back the issuance of social equity licenses have been settled or struck down, the first of the social equity licensees have opened, and there's a new energy in the air. People who have been patiently waiting to see minority-owned shops open are finally able to feel welcome in legal cannabis spaces. Chicago has yet to allow consumption lounges, but that—along with the lack of delivery options—is likely to change sooner rather than later. A new lay of the land is emerging, as the following pages will demonstrate, and Illinois cannabis is only going to get more interesting from here.

CHICAGO

CHICAGO

CHICAGO

LEGALIZED

Medical in 2013,
recreational in 2019

POSSESSION

Adults over the age of 21 can
possess: a little over an ounce
of cannabis flower, five grams
of concentrate, and up to five
hundred milligrams of THC in
a cannabis-infused product.
If you're from out of state, you
can purchase up to half of
these amounts.

HOME GROWS

You can grow up to
five cannabis plants
in your home.

DELIVERY

Not legal

CONSUMPTION

Smoking is allowed
on private property
or in permitted
spaces operated by
licensed cannabis or
tobacco retailers.

CITIES

Chicago

CHICAGO

CHICAGO

CHICAGO

DISPENSARY 33

ONE OF CHICAGO'S OLDEST LOCALLY OWNED AND COMMUNITY-ORIENTED CANNABIS SHOPS.

As the first medical shop in Chicago, Dispensary 33 is also ahead of the curve on design, creating a boutique space before anyone expected dispensaries to feel any different from a convenience store. Murals of seedlings and cannabis leaves are painted across the white walls, with items displayed from glass-topped, hexagonal cases in stylish clusters throughout the space. With the polished-but-approachable setting, the team here successfully struck a balance between a medical provider and a pleasant retail environment that's kept them one of the busiest shops in the state long after adult-use shops opened and big-chain dispensaries moved in.

They intentionally went for a slightly feminine design, aware that not everyone is into the average bro-oriented pot shop. The menu, however, appeals to everyone. I'd recommend checking out flower from local favorite Tales and Travels, delicious infused chocolate bars by family-owned brand Nature's Grace and Wellness, or any of the primo pre-rolls, sea salt caramels, and vape cartridges from Bedford Grow, one of the only independently run cannabis cultivators founded by Illinois natives.

Open Daily

**5001 N Clark Street
Chicago, IL 60640**

menu.dispensary33.com

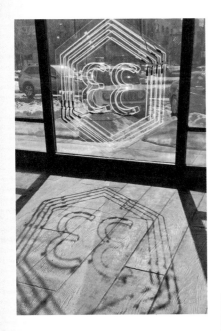

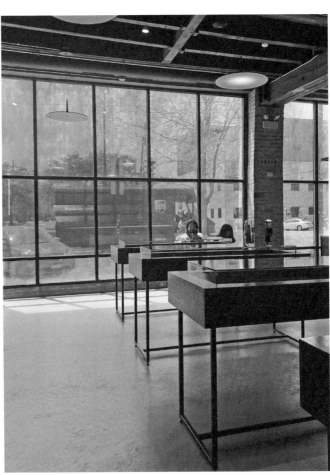

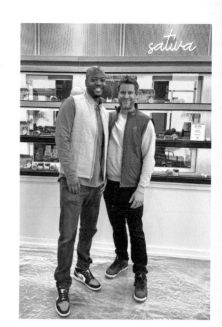

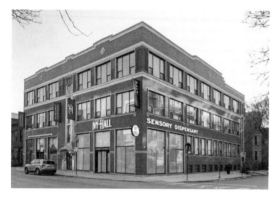

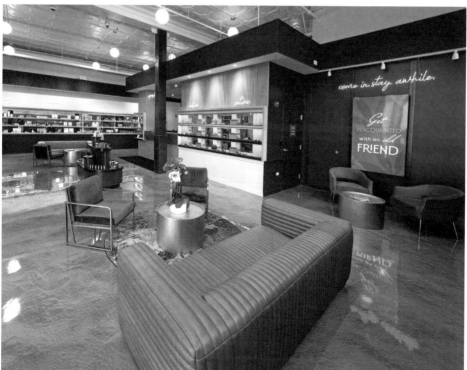

IVY HALL

A STYLISH, SENSORY, EQUITY-LICENSED DISPENSARY FOUNDED BY A PAIR OF CHICAGO NATIVES.

Few cannabis dispensaries embody the fusion of new and old like the pink neon accent lights reflecting off of the 130-year-old tin ceiling within Ivy Hall. The playful lighting is balanced with rich, emerald-toned walls and velvet chairs, cool marble floors, and lots of natural light from this stately historic building's tall windows. Ivy Hall is also home to a sensory bar, where guests can browse a collection of grab-n-smell jars of common cannabis aromas and terpenes, giving one a sample of the scent notes that can be found in the strains on the shelves.

Founders Nigel Dandridge and David Berger have been friends for over a decade, and have talked about running a weed store together for almost as long. Both born and raised in Chicago, they ended up eligible for one of the city's social equity licenses, making their dream possible. A couple of hard years later, their glamorous dispensary Ivy Hall opened its doors in the Bucktown neighborhood. In its name, Ivy represents the beauty of the natural world and the deep green color of cannabis, and they call it a hall because they hope for it to be a place where people gather to celebrate, communicate, and mark important points in history. Above all, Dandridge and Berger have high hopes that Chicagoans and all visitors will find that their ivy-hued haven is more than just a place to buy weed.

Open Daily

**1720 N Damen Avenue
Chicago, IL 60647**

ivyhalldispensary.com

WAKE-N-BAKERY

A QUIRKY NEIGHBORHOOD BAKE SHOP CELEBRATING SWEETS, TREATS, MULTICOLORED LEMONADES, AND ALL THINGS HEMP THC.

With the psychedelic paint job out front and the cannabis leaf-adorned signage overhead, the Wake-N-Bakery is a beacon for cannabis-friendly folk in Chicago's Lakeview neighborhood. Although you won't find real cannabis for sale here, you'll have the opportunity to carefully venture into the realm of delta-8 and delta-9 derived from hemp plants, and thus allowed to be sold outside of the state program. Delta-8 THC is just one chemical bond different from delta-9 and about a third to one half as potent. Because it technically comes from hemp, delta-8 and delta-9 have fallen under the generous, nearly totally unregulated hemp umbrella. For this reason, I am slow to recommend any product from this realm, and it's one that I always advise people to explore with the utmost caution.

Founder Brianna Banks was a former medical professional, and prior to opening the cafe, she and her business partner consulted lawyers, researched farms, and read through every legislation regarding hemp for months.

They set an age barrier of twenty-one for their baked goods and delta-8/9 drink infusions, and they have up-to-date certificates of analysis from third-party labs, which ensures there aren't any mold or toxic pesticides present in the hemp oil extract. Many come here because of a 2021 viral TikTok video that cemented their whimsical offerings in the internet's "weird, must-try food" section. The Strawberry Cough is one of their standbys: a house lemonade with strawberry puree, which you can have infused with a custom dose of hemp-derived THC. From the "Keep It Basic" base dose of thirty milligrams to the "Hell Yeah" dose of ninety milligrams, there's an infused treat for everybody. Fan favorites include their hemp THC-infused Rice Krispies treats and gluten-free blueberry scone —both priced at $4.20.

Open Daily

3508 N Broadway
Chicago, IL 60657

wakenbakery.net

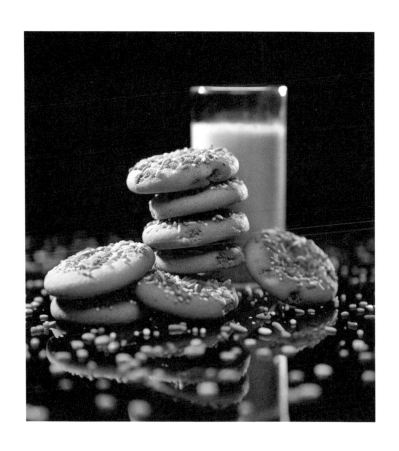

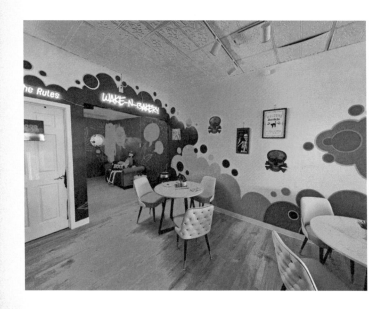

GRASSHOPPER CLUB

CHICAGO'S FIRST BLACK-OWNED CANNABIS DISPENSARY, REWRITING THE COMMUNITY'S RELATIONSHIP WITH WEED.

Perhaps it's the name, perhaps it's the original brick walls adorned with a mural by local graffiti calligraphy artist Tubsz, or maybe it's the retro memorabilia like a vintage bowling ball bag, an old-school pair of Jordan's, and a working turntable serving as décor. Whatever it is, there's something about Grasshopper Club that reminds me of a cannabis-themed HBCU fraternity from yesteryear. That isn't a real thing, of course, but that's kind of what co-founders Matthew Brewer, Chuck Brewer, and their mother, Dianne Brewer, intended to create: a space that celebrates the intertwined histories of Black culture and cannabis culture, Chicago legacy, and the passions and interests of the Brewer brothers—a passion that got Chuck arrested in his youth.

Between that past trauma and the long wait to open a shop in central Chicago, this shop means a great deal to the Brewers and the city's Black and Brown communities. When Grasshopper Club announced their opening date and started interviewing for staff, they received around one thousand applications for a mere twenty-five positions. The combination of a beautifully renovated historical space—located in the former Logan Square Trust & Savings Bank—a playful retro-meets-modern vibe, and a welcoming ambiance begs every guest to be their most unique selves as they comfortably shop in a space that dovetails from the typical overly sterile dispensary environments. Grasshopper Club also offers a thoughtfully curated menu, from Miss Grass pre-rolls to the Chicago native-grown flower from 93 Boyz, plus sought-after smoking accessories like Jane West glass and Rolling Rosa rolling papers.

Open Daily

**2551 N Milwaukee Avenue
Chicago, IL 60647**

grasshopperclub.com

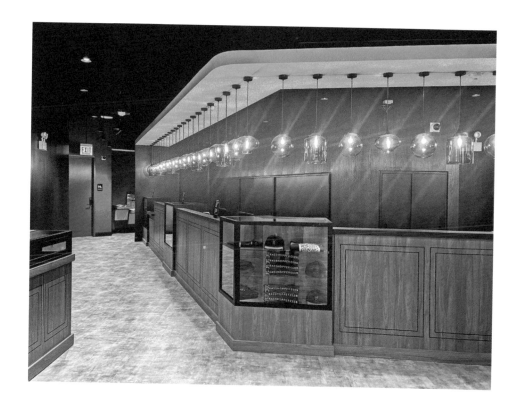

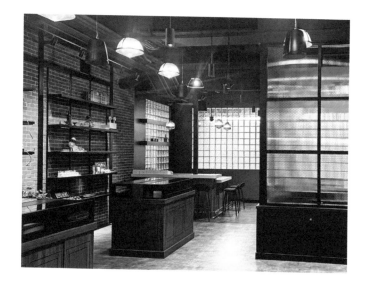

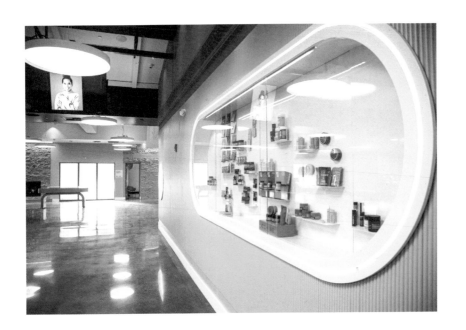

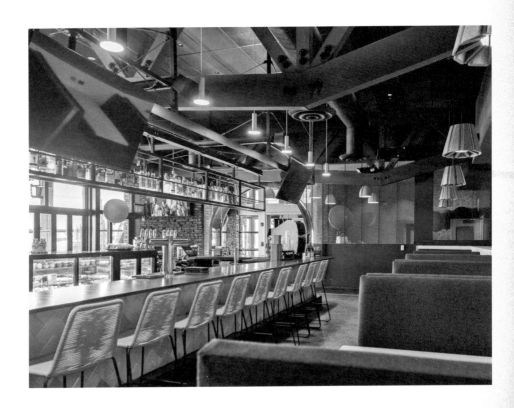

WEST TOWN BAKERY AND OKAY CANNABIS

A CAFE AND DISPENSARY SERVING CAKE BALLS, COCKTAILS, AND DANK CANNABIS UNDER ONE ROOF.

Imagine a true adult Candyland, where fresh, weed-free treats are served in the same space as infused gummies, chocolate bars, and alcoholic drinks, and you're in the ballpark of this West Town Bakery location that is conveniently connected to a fully licensed dispensary and a 100+-occupancy outdoor patio. It's a bright, colorful space with a playful vibe, perfectly separated by strategic spacing and ID checks to allow for a family-friendly bakeshop, a licensed bar, and a dispensary selling familiar flower, pre-rolls, gummies, topicals, and more to operate under one roof. Born from a collaboration between The Fifty/50 restaurant group and OKAY Cannabis, the space is designed to appeal to a range of people seeking a stimulating, fun environment—whether or not they intend to pick up fresh buds.

Maybe you're looking for an interesting date destination or a new environment to open up the laptop and catch up on emails, or maybe you're already a fan of master baker Chris Texeira's notoriously tasty pastries and artisan breads from one of the other West Town Bakery locations. Being able to get a nice, well-prepared latte made with locally roasted beans and a breakfast sandwich in the same building that I can grab a fresh eighth of flower is pretty much my dream wake-and-bake errand on a Saturday morning, and it's wildly impressive that the businesses were able to get a liquor license approved on the same site. This is what true normalization looks like. I'm so grateful that the city of Chicago is giving them a chance to prove that we, as cannabis consumers, can be responsible adults and handle these options without getting wildly intoxicated and burning the city down.

Open Daily

**781 N Milwaukee Avenue
Wheeling, IL 60090**

westtownbakery.com

HERBAL NOTES

A CHICAGO-BASED DINNER SERIES INFUSED WITH CANNABIS AND LATINO PRIDE, LED BY A MICHELIN-TRAINED CHEF.

You might recognize Manny Mendoza from an episode of Netflix's competitive cannabis cooking show, *Cooked With Cannabis.* He charmed the judges with leaf-shaped *chilaquiles* and infused *pupusas,* inspired by his time growing up immersed in Mexican and Salvadoran cuisine. A native of Chicago's Pilsen neighborhood, Mendoza's culinary path started at New York's Culinary Institute of America. After graduation, Mendoza was keen to start experimenting with cannabis infusions and happened to move back home just as the state was bringing their legal cannabis market online. While working at Owen & Engine and the Michelin-starred restaurant Senza, he began hosting private dinner parties, where attendees had the option of having their meal infused with a custom cannabis dose. Several years later, Mendoza has found a comfortable groove with his dinner series, Herbal Notes.

Every event is developed directly with the client, from menu details to infusion options. The experience itself can range from three to seven courses, and guests can choose whether they'd like a dropoff delivery or a full-service experience with Mendoza present. For new folks, he'll typically have everyone fill out a questionnaire before the dinners to get a sense of everyone's cannabis tolerance. He's a responsible chef, in that sense, but he's just as much a responsible cannabis advocate who's passionate about fostering positive cannabis experiences that break outdated stigmas.

In addition to his work as a chef, Mendoza is also an advisory board member for the Cannabis Equity Illinois Coalition, and through his creative menus, he's helping make the culinary cannabis space more welcoming to Latin flavors and ingredients, a community that has dealt with the negative associations of Reefer Madness for over a century. With Herbal Notes, Mendoza is offering a sensory combination of ancient ingredients and modern techniques that break the expectations of how cannabis can be consumed and brought into the mainstream. Take his spin on Quesadilla de la Milpa, made with Huitlacoche corn, mushroom, squash blossom, garden sofrito, and verdolagas (purslane) and assembled on a delicious homegrown and homemade cannabis tortilla.

**For event schedule, visit
herbalnotes.co/home**

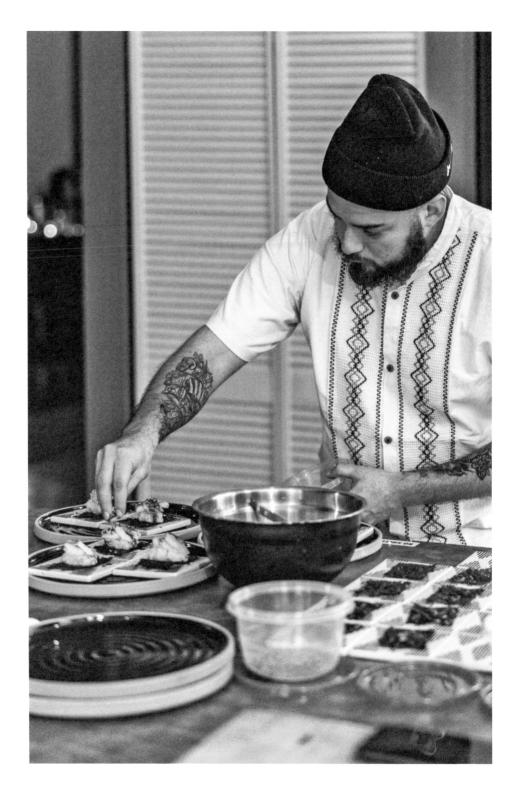

CHITIVA

A PAIR OF CANNABIS-ADJACENT HOTSPOTS SLINGING INFUSED SLUSHIES, HIGH-BROW PASTRIES, AND CHILL VIBES.

I'm in awe of Chitiva's creativity, and I'm not just talking about their homemade pints of precisely dosed, THC-infused ice cream or slushies. I'm talking about the clever legal savvy and out-of-the-box thinking that allows this business to legally provide cannabis-derived goods outside of the state's licensed dispensary program. Founder Charles Wu started Chitiva by providing farm tours in their state-of-the-art cultivation facility and developing into a retail concept that operates under the state's hemp regulation. The tours are no longer, but what came next proved that Wu's assessment of a few key loopholes in hemp and cannabis legislation were correct.

Technically, the flower they grow doesn't exceed the rules for THC content within the hemp regulations, and the oil they process to infuse into fresh-baked pastries, slushies, and ice cream offerings remain under the maximum milligrams of THC as well. Since they aren't a licensed dispensary, they are able to sell in-house flower and concentrates and host stoney yoga nights and vape-friendly bingo nights. Wu doesn't press his luck too far, though; both Chitiva locations are strictly twenty-one and up only, and everything containing any cannabinoids has been tested at the same certified third-party labs that licensed dispensaries are required to use. Wu and his team keep the majority of the supply chain in-house, allowing for eagle-eyed supervision and a consistency in quality that has built a lot of trust with the community very quickly.

In the summer, the frozen treats are a big draw, while James Beard Award-winning chef Steven Krizman has put the shops on the Chicago foodie map with his infused (and non-infused) pastries and fine desserts.

Open Tuesday–Sunday

**1948 W North Avenue
Chicago, IL 60622**

**For more locations, visit
chitiva.co**

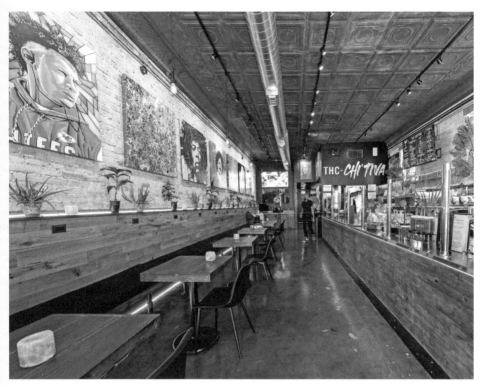

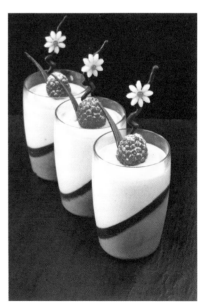

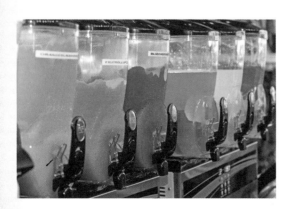

I've been a West Coast baby all of my life, but the first time I visited Detroit, Michigan, I felt something familiar. It certainly wasn't the demographic, as my home base in Portland is one of the least diverse cities in the country. No, it was the weed. It was the way it felt so comfortable to walk through downtown and catch a glimpse of the Detroit River while politely and somewhat discreetly smoking a joint. Without a doubt, this is the most cannabis-friendly state I've visited that doesn't border the Pacific Ocean (besides Colorado, I suppose). The long-established medical market has played a major role in the state of cannabis acceptance, and it continues to foster a community that cares deeply about the integrity of this plant. A quarter of a million folks—2.51 percent of the state's population—remained registered patients long after cannabis was legalized for all adults. Patient advocates have organized boycotts throughout the state—a rare occurrence in the exciting, celebratory environment of legal weed—and these boycotts actually made a difference, forcing many larger, publicly traded companies to play their cards wisely and partner with advocates to ensure their success.

While Detroit took its time to get adult-use stores up and operating, Ann Arbor is a different story. Home to the annual, unofficial cannabis festival Hash Bash, Ann Arbor decriminalized cannabis, to a degree, in the mid-1970s, and they're likely to be the first city in the state to decriminalize psilocybin, too. It's always been a progressive place, and one so locally minded that big publicly traded companies haven't really risked trying to compete with the small businesses that are already ingrained in the local cannabis community. In either city—across the state, really—there is a uniquely cannabis-forward energy to be found that every flower child ought to experience.

DETROIT   ANN ARBOR   DETROIT

LEGALIZED

Medical in 2008,
recreational in 2018

POSSESSION

Adults over the age of 21 can
possess: up to 2.5 ounces of
flower and fifteen grams of
concentrate, in oil or edible
form

HOME GROWS

Adults can grow up to
twelve cannabis plants
at home.

DELIVERY

Yes, but only to private
residences that match
the address on your
government-issued
ID (in other words:
locals only).

CONSUMPTION

Smoking is allowed on
private property or in
licensed consumption
spaces.

CITIES

Detroit
Ann Arbor

ANN ARBOR   DETROIT   ANN ARBO

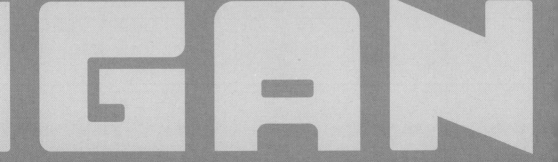

THE HIGH END AFFAIR

CELEBRITY CHEF NIKKI STEWARD'S NEXT-LEVEL CANNABIS DINNERS HOSTED THROUGHOUT THE MIDWEST AND BEYOND.

I should start by clarifying that Nikki Steward actually lives in Ohio. Her consistent culinary presence through her High End Affair infused dinners often take place in Detroit, which always trips me up, and I wouldn't be the first. In 2023, she was voted the people's choice for Best Cannabis Chef in Michigan by a landslide.

"Detroit is my second home—well, the whole Midwest is my home," Steward said. "But Detroit is a place that's really important to me. Not just the juxtaposition of demographics there, and that it's something like 80% Black and Brown, but also the legacy of dance here—the way people move."

To be clear, Steward isn't just a cannabis chef. For the past several years, she's been the go-to caterer for celebs like Dave Chapelle and Questlove, at one point touring with DJ Khaled to keep him, his crew, and select VIPs fed via a custom food truck that traveled from city to city. She still cooks for hire, but on the cannabis-infused side, she's grown more selective.

Over the past couple of years, the High End Affair has leaned into a High History concept—a riff on the *Drunk History* web series—starting with a series of dinners that educate attendees about the legacy of historic Detroit. She rented out three historic mansions in the city, one connected to the Kresge family (of Kmart fame) and another built by the Fisher family, and offered an infused spread of period-appropriate bites prepared by Steward and her all-women culinary team.

"It was just like what my grandmother would've cooked for a soiree in her twenties: oysters Rockefeller, canapes, deviled eggs, modernized ambrosia—all infused, but you could smoke or dab in the yard if preferred. I hired actors who dressed up as the historic figures and mingled with guests, and attendees dressed for a garden party dress code," Steward shared.

When we spoke, she was already planning another High History event in Detroit and New York, both more focused on the musical legacy of more recent decades. Tickets to these dinners aren't cheap, but you can expect a once-in-a-lifetime experience that will leave you well-fed and rich with new memories.

For event schedule, visit thehighendaffair.com

HOUSE OF ZEN

A LOW-KEY, SISTER-OWNED SHOP PROVIDING LOCALLY GROWN BUDS AND PERPETUALLY MELLOW VIBES.

After years of delays from social equity lawsuits in Detroit, Teri Hargrave and Jacqueline Weathersby's patience has paid off. The sisters were awarded the city's first adult-use retail license through the social equity program at the start of 2023 after operating House of Zen as a medical shop for several years, cultivating cannabis within the state's medical program. Both born and raised on Detroit's Eastside, they first got interested in the business of legal cannabis after seeing the relief Hargrave's husband experienced after using medical cannabis to treat his terminal lung cancer symptoms. He eventually passed away in 2014, inspiring his wife and her sister to create a safe, welcoming space for the community to congregate for plant medicine. It's a true family affair from the top down; when I called the shop on a Friday afternoon, I spoke with their nephew who was happily working as a budtender that day. I wouldn't mind working shifts at my family spot either if it had this kind of chill environment.

House of Zen is a little off the beaten path, located on a stretch that's home to a couple other dispensaries, so it never gets too crowded or noisy. The sisters wanted to design a space that reflected the calm feeling one gets from cannabis, using Eastern zen elements in the lobby to set the tone. They carry local favorites like small-batch flower from MJ Verdant and Goldkine, plus coveted vape cartridges by PC Pure, and a huge selection of smoking accessories from blunt wraps to mesh screens to keep those pesky bits from coming through your pipe's bowl.

Open Daily

14501 Mack Avenue
Detroit, MI 48215

houseofzendetroit.com

LIV CANNABIS DETROIT

A CENTRAL, THOUGHTFULLY DESIGNED, AND MINORITY-OWNED LOCAL DISPENSARY CHAIN.

The clean, sophisticated spaces of LIV Cannabis are actually operated by the Michigan-based company Common Citizen (CC), which acquired LIV in 2022. They're about as big as you can get while technically remaining a locally owned small business, but their largesse is what allows them to make a real difference: the founding team are all sons of immigrants who believe in their community and hire with intention.

Through a special partnership, LIV Cannabis' Detroit location is 51 percent owned by Black Detroiters. In all their stores, you'll find Principle, a pre-roll brand by CC, from which all of the profits go back to local community engagement and social equity programs in Detroit. Those programs, the partners they sent profits to, and other community initiatives are driven by their Director of External Affairs and Social Equity Jessica Jackson, who's also the co-founder of queer, cannabis-friendly bed-and-breakfast Copper House (see p. 196).

Open Daily

12604 E Jefferson Avenue
Detroit, MI 48215

For more locations, visit
livcannabis.com/detroit

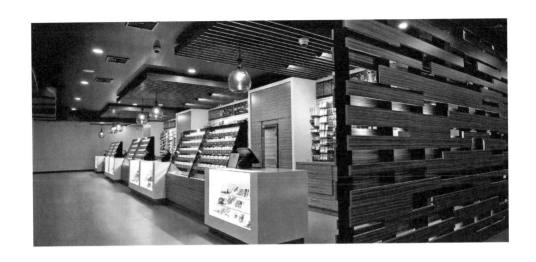

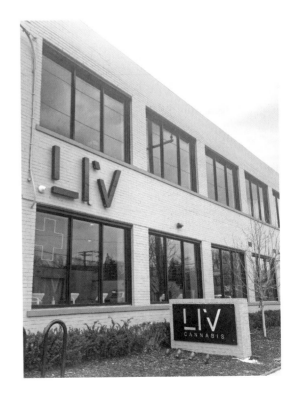

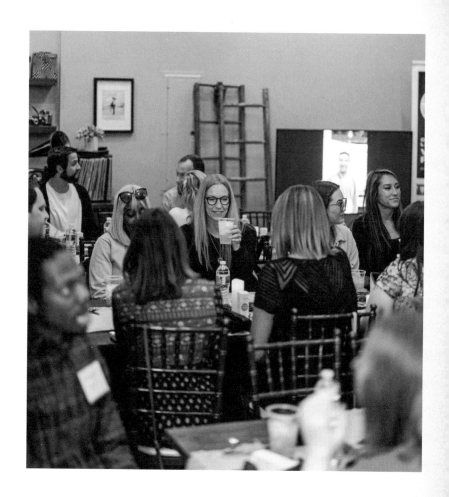

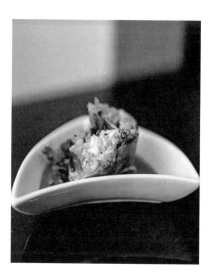

FALLING LEAVES EVENTS

A SOCIAL EQUITY-LICENSED CANNABIS EVENT COMPANY THAT FOSTERS CONNECTIONS FOR CANNABIS ENTREPRENEURS AND ENJOYERS THROUGHOUT DETROIT.

Every month of the year, Falling Leaves throws an event somewhere in the Detroit area. This steady, reliable cadence was a priority for founder and managing member Michael Webster, a longtime entrepreneur in the space who wants to help build community and break down stigmas around cannabis. Originally from New York, Webster's goal is to normalize cannabis in traditional spaces by promoting its mindful consumption in public to show people that it isn't any different than seeing someone sip a pint of beer. Falling Leaves is uniquely positioned to do this. With its state-issued cannabis event organizer license, they're allowed to have designated consumption and retail in the same space, which is super rare in the legislative landscape across the country. It also means they're required to keep up with very above-board elements like event insurance, which can run up to $10,000 for a one-day event.

The events started with a fine-dining approach geared toward industry folks looking to network and make deals over good food and flower. As the cannabis community evolved and Webster started to react to changing needs, he began offering more intimate dinners for cultivators to sponsor and make their own, providing a platform for emerging brands to create an experience and introduce themselves on their terms to their desired audience, be it dispensary buyers or local influencers.

Certain dinners will cater more to the public than others, with more of a self-serve vibe at some events to encourage mingling and interaction rather than settling into a clique at one end of the table. When there's likely to be more newbies in attendance, there is always a CBD station in the mix to help balance out anyone feeling too high. There's no shame in normalizing that, too. Just as folks are allowed to turn up at the club on a Saturday, it's OK to accidentally overdo it every now and again.

For event schedule, visit fallingleavesevents.com

LUCKY PISTIL CATERING

A BORN-AND-BRED DETROIT CHEF WHO IS RECLAIMING HER RELATIONSHIP TO CANNABIS THROUGH INFUSED CATERING.

Enid Parham did not grow up loving cannabis. In fact, she avoided it. Growing up as a Black woman in Detroit in the DARE era, Parham was conditioned to fear cannabis as a scary drug that would only bring harm. It wasn't until the difficulties she experienced following the loss of her father that she opened her mind to alternative methods to manage her anxiety. Weed helped her sleep and find happiness— two things she desperately needed while navigating grief as a single mom. The plant medicine made her feel so much clearer than prescription pills, and she felt more capable of re-entering social life. All of this transformed her perspective on this plant and plant medicine in general.

At the time, she was working at the Ritz Carlton and started to hear stories from the West Coast about infused dinner parties and culinary pop-ups. She looked up recipes to try making her first batch of weed butter, and in no time she was hosting private brunches in a downtown Detroit space, topping savories and sweets with infused butter. Over time, those brunches became intimate dinners with handwritten invitations complete with a secret code to access the unlisted location, and soon, Parham found herself running one of the city's first underground supper clubs. Once legal sales in Michigan kicked off, Parham decided to make things official. She named the project after her favorite part of the plant and the act of taking her destiny into her own hands.

"If I make it, I'm lucky," Parham said in a past interview with me. "So I'm the Lucky Pistil."

She also goes by Chef Sunflower, which makes sense if you get the fortune of sitting at her table. Parham has a radiant, welcoming energy and adds an air of humble gratitude into everything she does.

For event schedule, visit luckypistil.com

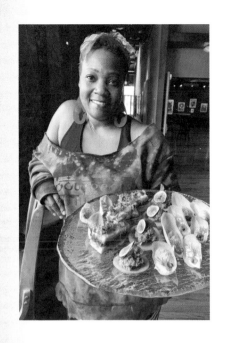

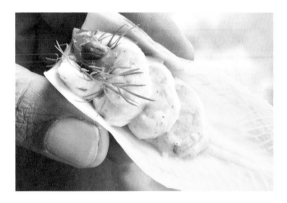

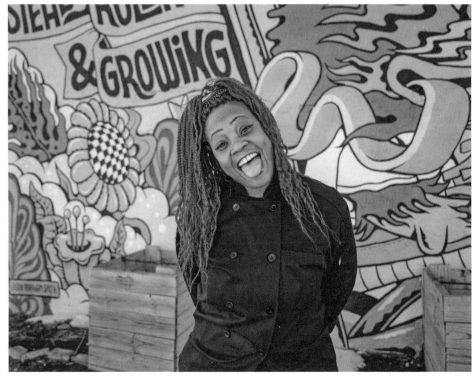

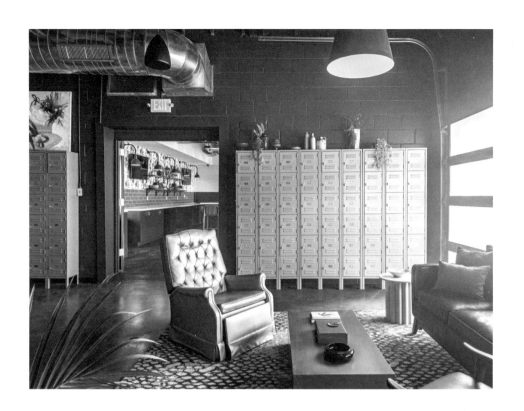

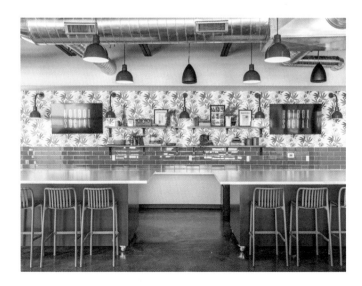

HOT BOX SOCIAL

A WELL-APPOINTED, LICENSED CONSUMPTION LOUNGE WITH A TROPICAL BAR VIBE ON THE NORTH END OF DETROIT.

Although there's no alcohol in sight at Hot Box Social, the very cute, emerald green and light pink color palette make his spot feel like a tropical bar, giving every corner of this space a selfie-ready vibe. Rest assured, though, there are plenty of cannabis products brought from home or delivered by Hot Box's partner Breeze for folks to choose from. It's a playful, social atmosphere that feels like a hot new date night spot in town, but in actuality it's one of the more established consumption lounges in this part of the country. That clean, professional, and thoughtfully designed approach is likely what's kept this spot at the top of the game over the course of the COVID-19 pandemic.

Located in a restored Thunderbird repair shop, there is a main lounge, a more intimate "Hot Box Room," and a back patio, providing ample room for events like *RuPaul's Drag Race* viewing parties and expungement clinics alongside regulars just seeking a chill, emerald velvet couch upon which to leisurely enjoy a joint. This is a bring-your-own-cannabis-and-accesories kind of joint, so be sure to bring whatever you need for the perfect smoke sesh.

Besides weed, though, there are plenty of reasons to swing by that won't require any accessories, from infused dining experiences and even black tie fundraisers for cannabis-related startups. Hot Box Social is exactly how it sounds: a place you can be social, hot box with strangers and friends, and host whatever kind of cannabis-friendly event the community needs.

Open Monday & Tuesday & By Appointment

**23610 John R Road
Hazel Park, MI 48030**

hotboxsocial.us

JESSICA JACKSON, CO-FOUNDER OF COPPER HOUSE, A CANNABIS-FRIENDLY BED-AND-BREAKFAST AND EVENT SPACE CATERING TO QUEER WOMEN

copperhousedet.com

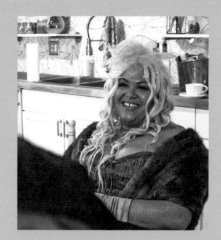

To me, Detroit natives Jessica and Jacqara Jackson are the epitome of creative cannabis entrepreneurs. They founded Copper House because of their own experiences while traveling abroad. Even in the red light district of Amsterdam, it's not easy to find a cannabis consumption-friendly lodging that also feels safe and welcoming to queer people, particularly queer women. So, when Michigan legalized cannabis for adult use in 2018, just a few months after they'd become the proud owners of a large, historic house with a spare bedroom in the Bagley neighborhood, a light bulb sparked. In January 2019, their first guest made their reservation at Copper House—named for Jess and Jacqara's collection of copper pieces displayed throughout the house. Over time, the space became more than just an Airbnb or a cannabis-friendly venue; it became a hub for Detroit's growing cannabis scene. Jessica now juggles her role as Common Citizen's director of external affairs and social equity with Copper House operations and ongoing advocacy, and remains a ray of comforting light when you get the privilege of meeting her in person. In this conversation with Jessica, we chatted about a major renovation at Copper House, the state of equity in cannabis, and her dreams for the Michigan cannabis scene.

WHAT'S THE LATEST AT COPPER HOUSE?

We now have a full one-thousand-square-feet studio apartment with a kitchenette available to guests, the renovation of which was largely funded through a donation from the nonprofit Cannabis for Black Lives. People continue to use the space to curate events, use it as a photo studio, pop up a massage event, or even a podcast recording sesh. We try to maintain a 60/40 ratio with events and overnight booking. It's still a residential environment; we don't want to become a venue. With the larger space, we're pushing "potjama" parties and bachelorette parties, and we've added accessories like a gravity bong and an Ardent machine for making your own edibles. It's been powerful to see what it can mean to not just provide a safe space, but really hold space for the community. During Pride celebrations each year, we go big. We hosted a Christmas drive last year, gathering donations for gifts and volunteers to gift wrap, and we ended up providing gifts for five families negatively impacted by the War on Drugs.

HOW DO YOU DESCRIBE DETROIT'S WEED SCENE?

I'd say there are a few different buckets of cannabis communities right now. There are the patient and caregiver advocates of the established medical industry who care deeply about patients' rights to access affordable, quality medicine. Then, there's the classic stoner community, which is organizing its own gray-area events. There are these underground trade shows where people who prefer buying straight from legacy growers can do so. High-quality products can be found in the legacy market, and some people don't feel comfortable walking into dispensaries that feel like an Apple Store.

WHAT ARE YOUR HOPES FOR THE MICHIGAN MARKET?

I hope that more than just reinvesting financially, we work toward ways that add value to minority communities. Beyond charitable donations, I want to see diverse suppliers within operations. Who are you paying for internet? Tech assistance? Packaging services? There are so many ways to contribute to a more equitable industry, and it's more accessible to small businesses to opt for sustainable and easily implemented support like these. I hope to keep seeing new ideas germinate at Copper House as well. A large part of what I want to do with Copper House is inspire other people to stake their claim with whatever they have. I had a house, so I figured out how to make it an asset and add value to it.

There's one woman throwing monthly educational tea parties here, and she has grown to hundreds of followers. She's about to outgrow the space, and I couldn't be happier. That's my ultimate goal.

INFORMATION ENTROPY

A PAIR OF HIGH-DESIGN DISPENSARIES LOCATED IN HISTORIC BUILDINGS AND STOCKED WITH BELOVED HOUSE FLOWER AND HASH.

When driving down Broadway, locals and visiting tourists alike still do a double take at the renovated church with the obscure name. Is it the home base of a New Age religion? A third-wave cafe? The answer is clear the minute one actually opens the front door, and the slight aroma of fresh, fire cannabis flower hits your nostrils. This location is a former church, in fact one that was originally built in the 1800s. The crisp white interiors maintain a holy atmosphere, though, with dark wood floors and polished display shelves that present the available strains with a special kind of reverence. The family-owned store is a trusted destination for flower and strain-specific concentrate, from their exclusive house buds to a range of hash rosin cartridges processed from that flower.

Founder Drew Hutton was born and raised in Ann Arbor, which is another reason many locally driven Ann Arborans will seek out one of Information Entropy's locations. At both spots, you can expect experienced service from budtenders that have all worked elsewhere in the industry before joining the IE team. Folks are encouraged to take the flower display samples into their own hands and smell them for reference, and if it's clear they truly care about shopping by aroma, budtenders will happily bust out bigger bags of each strain for a more encompassing whiff.

About that name: Hutton has a degree in mathematics and economics from University of Michigan, and he named the business after a concept within the study of "information theory." I do not understand what any of that means, but I love the authentic math nerd inspo behind it.

Open Daily

1115 Broadway Street
Ann Arbor, MI 48105

For more locations, visit
informationentrophy.com

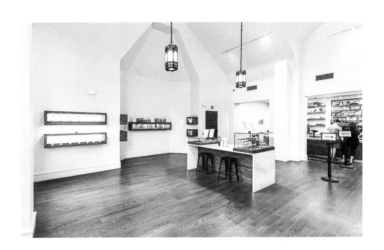

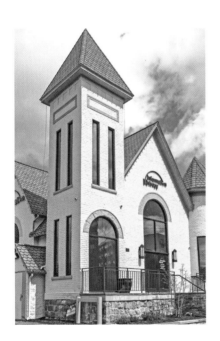

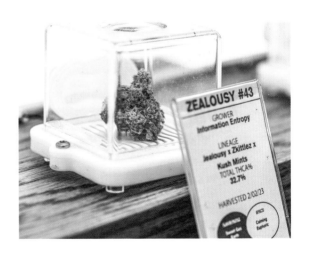

ZEALOUSY #43

GROWER
Information Entropy

LINEAGE
Jealousy x Zkittlez x
Kush Mints
TOTAL THCA%
32.7%

HARVESTED 2/02/23

Calming
Euphoric

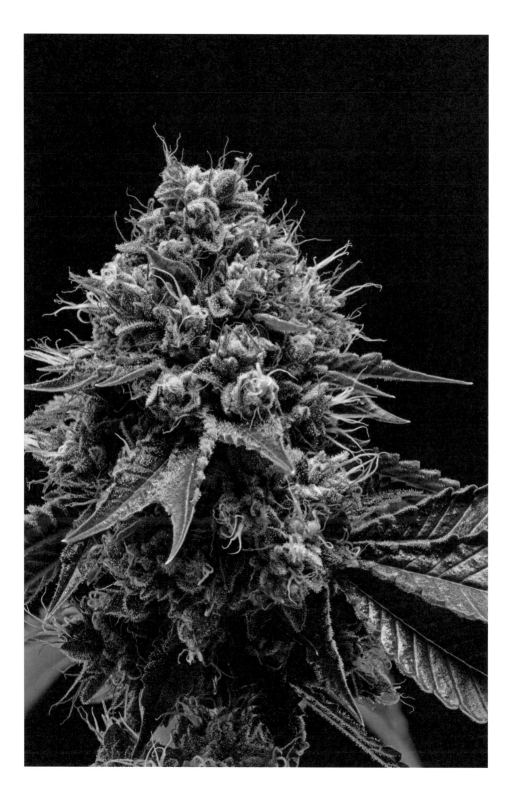

WINEWOOD ORGANICS

A COZY MINI DISPENSARY WITH AN EQUALLY COZY SELECTION OF HOUSE-GROWN FLOWER.

Like many West Coast weed lovers, I have an uncle or two with a Boomer-tastic smoking pad in their garage—forty-year-old couch, sixty-year-old ashtrays, and an ambient layer of dust (and nostalgic charm), no matter how recently it's been cleaned. Winewood Organics is what I imagine a more feminine sesh area curated by a cool hippie aunt would look and feel like.

Houseplants and Persian rugs lend a welcoming living room feel, and as a "microbusiness," it is actually not a whole lot bigger than the average living room. The family-run shop intentionally aimed for an earthy, relaxing vibe, avoiding the path toward the Apple Store energy that many modern dispensaries have followed. There is only one brand of cannabis, concentrates, resin cartridges, fruit gummies, and chocolates on the shelves, and that's Winewood Organics, which is a very unique approach that I find particularly intriguing. This is a shop actively going against the more-is-more mentality and standing by their house flower in a way that says a great deal about their faith in its quality.

Open Daily

2394 Winewood Avenue
Ann Arbor, MI 48103

winewoodorganics.com

THE REFINERY

A TRUSTWORTHY WESTERN MICHIGAN DISPENSARY CHAIN FOUNDED BY PASSIONATE CULTIVATORS STOCKING STATEWIDE FAVORITES.

As a regular consumer and, dare I say, "cannabis connoisseur," there's no single dispensary in my area that satisfies all my needs. I most frequently swing by a couple no-frills neighborhood shops that always have fresh flower in stock from my favorite growers, but if friends or family are visiting from out-of-town, we'll head over to one of the more posh spots with well-designed interiors for "oohs" and "aahs." Then there's the spot with the biggest selection of low-dose edibles that I like to hit up on the way to dinner with my grandmother.

The Refinery's locations in Kalamazoo and Traverse City aren't necessarily gunning for *Architectural Digest* mentions, but they are by far the most frequently recommended stops by budget-minded connoisseurs and the daily dabbers in town for the weekend. Founded by a group of West Michigan-based growers, every product stocked is vetted by their high—and very experienced—standards.

And, boy, are there a lot of products here. Trending strains, hype new gummy brands, novel disposable vaporizers and cartridges—this is where you go when your stash is low and you don't want to be disappointed. I should clarify that while they didn't go the white Carrara marble countertop route, the space is still clean, professional, fun, and staffed with knowledgeable folks who care about helping you find exactly what you're looking for.

Open Daily

3650 Alvan Road
Kalamazoo, MI 49001

For more locations, visit
refinemi.com

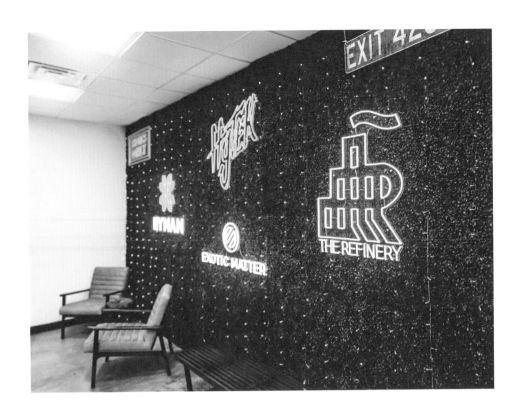

MI 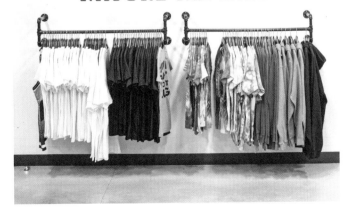 US

THE REFINERY
NATURE REFINED

MASSACHUSETTS   NEW JERSEY   N

E   A

RSEY   NEW YORK   VERMONT   M

COAST

NT   MAINE   MASSACHUSETTS   NE

HUSETTS   NEW JERSEY   NEW YORK   VE

VERMONT

MAINE

MASSAC

S

T

MASSACHUSETTS

NEW JERSEY

NEW YOR

NEW YORK

NE

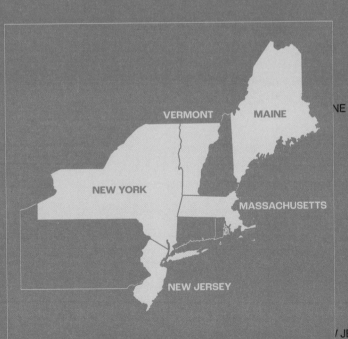

VERMONT   MAINE

NEW YORK

MASSACHUSETTS

NEW JERSEY

MAINE

/ JEI

Maine is the cannabis-cultivation capital of the East Coast. Many New England operators I spoke to that had worked all over made the argument that Maine is home to the best concentrates and—depending on the strain—the best flower in the country. Even those living in neighboring states where cannabis is legal will make the drive across the border for some locally grown goodness. There is a craft cultivation scene here that seems to stand a head above the rest, largely populated by small growers who care deeply about the way they grow the flower they provide to dispensaries. The twenty-five-year-old medical market has been largely populated by small boutique farms differentiated by unique strains and impeccable cultivation practices. There's a long history of cannabis and hash competitions, unofficial 4/20 pot holiday gatherings, and a lack of dirty looks if you happen to smell extra fragrant when sitting down to enjoy some fresh-caught lobster.

Not-so-hidden gems abound in this intimate cannabis community and the equally intriguing food scene. In fact, *Bon Appetit* magazine named Portland the Restaurant City of the Year in 2018, and Biddeford was selected as one of America's next great food cities in 2022 by *Food & Wine*. While many come for the seafood, it's becoming a destination for vegetarians, vegans, and, of course, flower children like me who are interested in the *other* local greens.

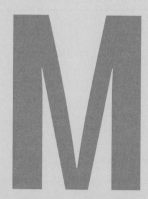
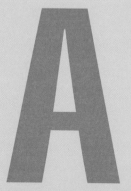

LEGALIZED

Medical in 1999,
recreational in 2016

POSSESSION

Adults over the age of
21 can possess: 2.5
ounces of a combination
of cannabis, cannabis
concentrate, and
cannabis products,
including no more than
five grams of cannabis
concentrate

HOME GROWS

Adults can grow three
mature plants, twelve
immature plants, and
as many seedlings as
they'd like.

DELIVERY

Yes, but only to private
residences (no hotels).

CONSUMPTION

Smoking is allowed on
private property.

CITIES

Portland

PORTLAND   PORTLAND   PORTLAN▸

I   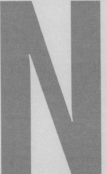   E

MEOWY JANE

A CAT-THEMED BOUTIQUE AND DISPENSARY LOCATED IN CHARMING, WALKABLE OLD PORT.

People told Noelle Albert that it wasn't a good idea to name her medical marijuana dispensary after a cat pun, but she did it anyway, and she leaned all the way in. In this quirky shop, there are fake robo-kitties that move and purr, and there is more than one cat-themed ashtray on display. The Meowy Jane team also partners with shelters to host cat adoption events (at which most cats end up getting adopted). While some folks do come in assuming it's some kind of cat cafe, most are intrigued to sit down and chat awhile, put at ease by the charming, airy space.

As a previously licensed medical shop, Meowy Jane was grandfathered into the adult-use system; however, due to Maine's cannabis laws, their house flower hasn't been able to hit the shelves just yet. A longtime cultivator, Albert is looking forward to it, but for now, she's got plenty of trustworthy farms and producers she's proud to recommend. She says edibles are the top seller for them, with many customers opting for the ease and fast-acting effects of infused drinks. The Hashery's hash rosin-infused drinks can also be found here, as well as truly fresh-baked edibles from local brand Pot & Pan.

Even if you aren't craving any cannabinoids, this is a great spot to stock up on solid smoking accessories, too. You can find pieces by GRAV, a reliable name that does simple, everyday glass pieces perfectly, as well as dainty, ornamental porcelain bongs by vintage refurbisher My Bud Vases. There's also jewelry by local artists, indie magazines (yes, *Broccoli*'s in the house), CBD intimacy oil by East Coast favorite Citrine, and a generally dreamy aesthetic that's perfect for capturing any cat mom/stoner girl content.

Open Daily

**3 Market Street
Portland, ME 04101**

meowyjane.org

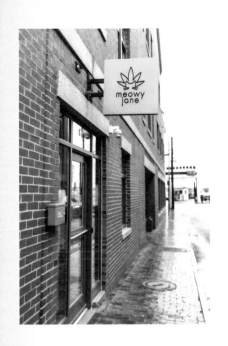

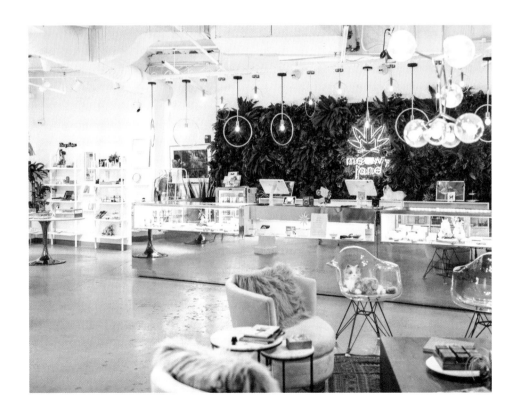

HAZY HILL FARM

A LEADING CULTIVATOR IN THE MAINE SCENE AND A DESTINATION DISPENSARY FOR CONCENTRATE CONNOISSEURS.

Once my research got underway and I made contact with the cultivators and cannabis chefs in each region, this guide (sort of) started writing itself. Hazy Hill Farm was one of those spots that wasn't on my radar until I had cracked into the New England weed community, and, once I had, I learned even the most connected people in Massachusetts and Connecticut's legal markets make time to drive over to this simple, streamlined shop when their stash runs low.

The homegrown flower here is phenomenal, cultivated by locals who have operated in the medical program for over a decade and care deeply about delivering high-quality, high-impact flower and live hash rosin

pressed by esteemed craft processors. On the edibles side, expect interesting finds like hash rosin peanut butter cups by High Peak and Rock City Coffee by Highbrow, a line of decaf, full-body grounds infused with THC distillate for a soothing cup of fresh-brewed coffee you can make at home. Hazy Hill Farm is the kind of place with such high standards that even if whatever strain you saw online ran out by the time you arrived, you can trust anything else you try will be safe, fresh, delicious, and potent.

Open Daily

484 Congress Street
Portland, ME 04101

hazyhillfarm.com

FIRE ON FORE

A SWAG-FILLED, CONNOISSEUR-APPROVED DISPENSARY IN THE MIDDLE OF THE COBBLESTONE STREETS OF HISTORIC OLD PORT.

This was another one of the flower-forward spots highly recommended to me from connoisseurs all over the Northeast. I'd overlooked it at first because, like most restaurants, cafes, and sights to see in tourist trap historical districts, I assumed it'd serve overpriced, subpar goods. But that is not the case for the aptly named Fire on Fore, which actually got voted the people's favorite dispensary in a 2023 regional poll.

Here you can find many of this state's finest farms under one roof—Firefly Organics, Hazy Hill Farm, Kind & Co., and Calendar Islands Cannabis, to name a few. There are dozens of options for concentrates and disposable vaporizers, too, plus tasty and portable edible options like potent syrups by Squier's Specialty Edibles and lower-dose canned drinks by Wynk. If you're in town for a visit and are looking for memorabilia while in this historical district, purchase some of their swag. They offer a vast selection of equally fire smoking accessories and apparel, with really cool limited drops of tees and hoodies printed with strain-inspired designs and even branded boxers.

Open Daily

367 Fore Street
Portland, ME 04101

fireonfore.com

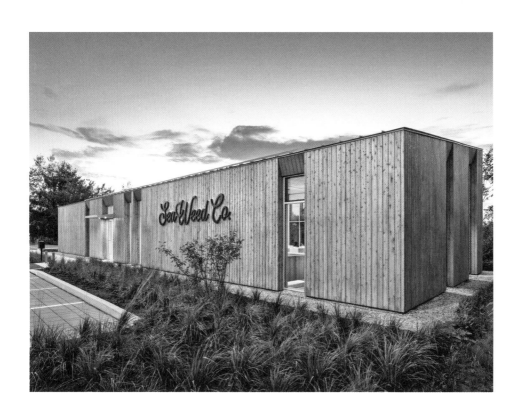

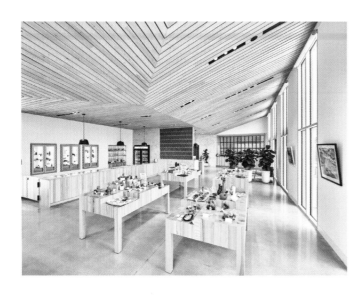

SEAWEED CO.

A PAIR OF SEA-INSPIRED, TRANSPORTIVE DISPENSARIES THAT CELEBRATE PORTLAND'S MAKERS AND CULTIVATORS.

Founded by avid fisherman and fly fishing guide, Scott Howard, the theme at the charming and aesthetically pleasing SeaWeed Co. is none other than the ocean. Budtenders are "mermaids" here, and the wooden exterior of the building looks like it was built by found driftwood. Inside, it's more like Ariel's dream boutique, where fine flower, finer vape cartridges, and all kinds of locally made art and home goods can be found.

At the flagship location in South Portland, you can find potted succulents and houseplants, ceramics, artful vases, leather goods, hemp CBD treats for humans and pets, and a similar spread of non-cannabis offerings. This bright, beautifully designed space is the kind of shop that plenty of people bring their friends and family to in order to help break their past stigmas about cannabis. Howard also has a manufacturing facility where his team processes their own concentrates that are sold all over the state. These strain-specific live resin cartridges, dab-ready concentrates, and edibles sell fast, though, so if you want

to be sure they're in stock, it's best to head to one of their Portland home bases.

They have long worked with trusted farms like Grass Roots, Divine Buds, and Gėlė for their raw plant product, and both the SeaWeed Co. processors and in-house "mermaids" appreciate the nuance of quality cannabis products. Rather than organizing the shop menu by the essentially made up terms of indica and sativa or the THC content—one indicator among many that determine a strain's effects—products are arranged by dominant terpene. It inspires more conversation between customers and staff, and gives folks a clearer understanding of the science behind how this plant makes us feel.

Open Daily

185 Running Hill Road
South Portland, ME 04106

For more locations, visit
seaweedmaine.com

HIGHER GROUNDS

A FULL-SERVICE CBD CAFE OFFERING HEMP-INFUSED LATTES, UNINFUSED BAKED GOODS, AND REAL MEDICAL CANNABIS.

You could consider Higher Grounds a well-stocked hemp dispensary that includes a cafe and, if you're a certified patient in Maine's medical program, a real weed menu. I consider it a brilliant, highly accessible way to help people understand the many reasons people turn to hemp and cannabis. When you walk in, it looks like any other chill, plant-filled, third-wave café. That is until the barista asks if you have a medical card. If so, they'll gesture you toward the dispensary part of the space, and, if not, you'll stroll up to make your coffee order or shop their hemp-derived offerings. It's a pleasant enough space that many come here just to open up their laptop and kick back for a few hours, as they would in any cafe.

They have a hyper-local eye when stocking their shelves, prominently featuring full-spectrum CBD salves, tinctures, vapes, and certified organic, Maine-grown hemp flower from Rooted Heart Remedies and Mindful Earth. It's not easy to find well-grown hemp pre-rolls online, but all the hemp and cannabis products here are grown in this state. Higher Grounds may not yet offer full-on cannabis to all who enter, but it's a founding member of the Maine Craft Cannabis Association—a group of independent cannabis businesses, advocates, and enthusiasts fighting for fair, local, and craft-oriented cannabis policy—and has a nurse practitioner on staff to offer guidance to any inquiring patients.

Open Daily

45 Wharf Street
Portland, ME 04101

highergrounds.me

STONER & CO.

A UNIQUE DISPENSARY FOUNDED BY STONERS, FOR STONERS INTERESTED IN CAREFULLY CULTIVATED HOUSE FLOWER.

Located in a small town just south of Portland, this shop is a labor of love for Morgan and Karleena Stoner (yes, that's their real last name). The couple met in 1992, married in 2014, and started Stoner & Co. together in 2015. The store's modern gothic aesthetic is a playful springboard for the names of their strains and products, essentially all of which are grown and produced in-house.

All of the craft flower and pre-rolls are grown by the Stoners (I love how that sounds!), and the concentrates are made from their flower and processed by East Coast Cannabis. There's even a balanced, 1:1 chocolate bar infused with house flower on the menu, a square of which is, in my opinion, the ideal anti-anxiety dose—and house-made tinctures. They also carry sour gummies from Glaze and low-dose infused seltzers by Calm Springs, but it's about quality over quantity here. In my research, people loved their flower, but they especially loved the good energy they felt upon walking into the shop. It's a cool space with an old-timey feel that lends well to a range of fun, branded accessories and a helpful, educated staff that knows these products inside and out.

Open Daily

414 Hill Street
Biddeford, ME 04005

stonerandco.com

The East Coast's green wave of state legalization started here in Massachusetts, where cannabis has increasingly become a part of the social lives of locals. There are, truly, some of the most architecturally stunning dispensaries in the country in the Great Barrington region and a notable number of infused culinary experiences popping up in Boston, even a hemp-infused meal kit service called Dinner at Mary's. Considering time-honored cannabis celebrations like the Boston Freedom Rally, where thousands gather on the Boston Common on the third Saturday in September for a hazy protest of pot prohibition, this state's been primed for a dynamic scene to establish for a while now.

Regulations were ahead of the curve here as well, with early plans to pardon past nonviolent, cannabis-related offenses and expunge charges for crimes that, today, would be considered legal. The state is still ironing out the kinks in its cannabis program, as all states are, but there's a passionate push for locally owned operators to see "Mass Proud" small businesses survive and thrive. There's a cap to how many shops a brand can have, so no one can be the CVS of weed here. This has fostered a lot of shops with personality and interesting products and encouraged business owners to try out new approaches. Without a doubt, Massachusetts is a scene to watch.

GREAT BARRINGTON   BOSTON   WORCESTER   MARTHA'S VINEYAR

MASSAC

LEGALIZED

Medical in 2012,
recreational in 2016

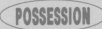 **POSSESSION**

Adults over the age of 21
can possess: one ounce
of flower, five grams
of concentrates, five
hundred milligrams of
edibles, or five thousand
milligrams of tincture

HOME GROWS

Adults can grow up to
six plants.

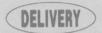 **DELIVERY**

Yes, but only to private
residences (no hotels).

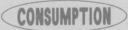 **CONSUMPTION**

Smoking is allowed on
private property.

 CITIES

Great Barrington
Boston
Worcester
Martha's Vineyard

GREAT BARRINGTON   BOSTON   WORCESTER   MARTHA'S VINEYAR

HUSETTS

FARNSWORTH FINE CANNABIS

AN ARCHITECTURALLY STUNNING DISPENSARY WITH A LEGACY OF AMERICAN INNOVATION ENTRENCHED IN ITS DNA.

It hurts me to say it, but when it comes to high-design dispensaries, there are few shops on the West Coast that can hold a torch to this little gem nestled in the highlands of Massachusetts. Farnsworth Fine Cannabis is a creation from fashion designer Adam Lippes and brothers Alexander and Brayden Farnsworth, featuring interiors designed by London-based architect Simon Aldridge and inspired by the grand shapes of Rome's arched Colosseo Quadrato.

Gold-leaf art sculptures gleam from various corners of the bright, two-thousand-square-foot space. The house pre-rolls are whole-flower "cannabis cigarettes," containing aromatic ground buds rather than the powdery shake that sometimes fills the more affordable options and cleanly, chicly packaged like a box of actual designer cigarettes. Farnsworth Fine Cannabis carries other Massachusetts brands like flower from Nature's Heritage, CANN's infused sparkling drinks, as well as house flower, edibles, and sensual body oil.

Besides cannabis consumables, there are premium flower grinders and heavy-duty glass smoking accessories from Higher Standards on the beautifully backlit shelves, plus a fabulous collection of vintage radios that happen to include one with the brand name "Farnsworth." Alexander and Brayden's great-great uncle, Philo Farnsworth, was an inventor, and not just any inventor; he invented the electronic television. He never saw a fortune from his invention (his patent ran out before it generated any riches), but if Farnsworth Fine Cannabis continues to provide such a must-see, high-quality cannabis experience, both atmospherically and flower-wise, the family name just might see those fortunes after all.

Open Daily

126 Main Street
Great Barrington, MA 01230

farnsworthfinecannabis.com

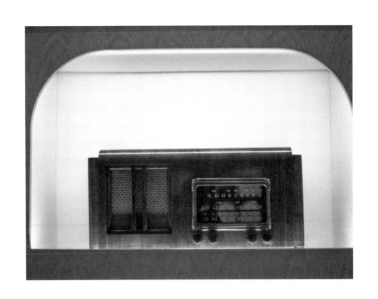

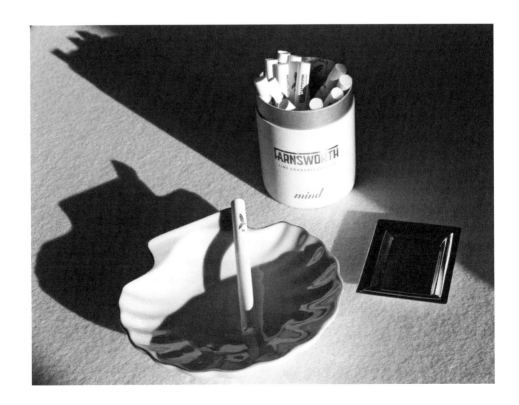

REBELLE

A WOMEN-RUN SHOP WITH BEAUTIFUL INTERIORS AND EQUALLY BEAUTIFUL ARTISAN ACCESSORIES.

Founded by a New York-based trio of friends and entrepreneurs Charlotte Hanna, Geraldine Hessler, and Penelope Nam-Stephen, Rebelle is a beautiful shop that reflects an equally thoughtful effort toward building a more equitable industry. They work with nonprofit Roca to recruit new interns and staff members from communities like Pittsfield and North Adams that have been hurt by the criminalization of cannabis, plus they contribute to an expungement fund on an ongoing basis to help eligible people overturn low-level cannabis convictions in Massachusetts. They also didn't skimp on design, creating a sophisticated, minimalist space that highlights their high-brow selection of interesting products and smoking accessories.

You can pick up patterned rolling papers and luxury leather stash bags here, peruse Session Goods' award-winning bongs and pipes, and ogle at their fantastic selection of handheld vapes that you can fill with your desired concentrate. There are the familiar

PAX devices, curated pieces from niche brands like Vessel, and a variety of e-rigs for aspirational dabbers by Puffco. Among the curated dozen or so flower strains and pre-roll varieties, they also offer fresh buds from Nature's Heritage, a farm I've heard East Coast cannabis folks speak highly of for years. The modest assortment of concentrates include rosin from local favorite Blue River and a rich topical balm by SLATE containing the perfect balance of THC and CBD that works great to help muscles repair after strain.

Don't miss out on the house offerings, which includes a very cool, high-tech edible product line called HALØ that produces a collection of 0.5- to 1-milligram THC "microdosing mists," infused mouth sprays with other beneficial compounds like green tea extract and chlorophyll.

Open Daily

783 S Main Street
Great Barrington, MA 01230

letsrebelle.com

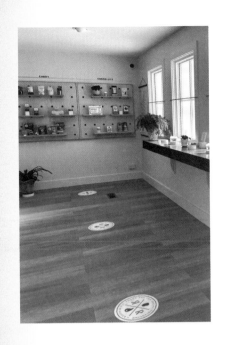

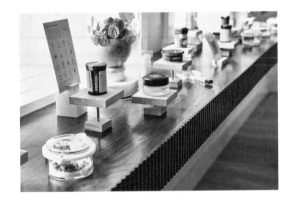

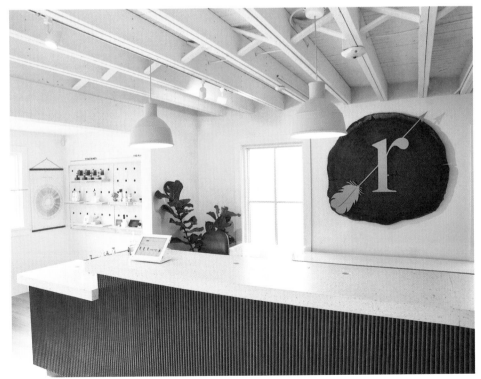

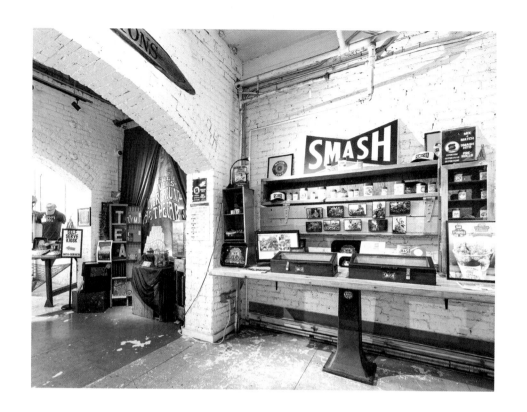

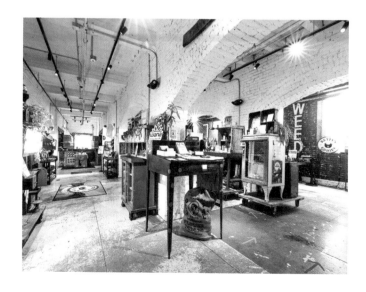

CANNA PROVISIONS

A LOCAL CHAIN WITH CHARMING, VINTAGE SENTIMENTS AND A LEGIT ASSORTMENT OF OLD-SCHOOL STRAINS.

You know those classic strain names of yore like Acapulco Gold and Maui Wowie? Even if you see those 1970s-80s era names on shelves, chances are those strains will taste and feel nothing like the Maui Wowie or AC that my parents sparked up back in the day. That's because during the height of the War on Drugs, the majority of those classic plants got flushed down the toilet or burned up during raids. And that's why it's very, *very* cool that the OG cut of the beloved Chemdog strain can be found at Canna Provisions and *only* Canna Provisions.

Greg "Chemdog" Krzanowski is their director of cultivations, bringing with him plants that he's cultivated since the 1990s. This particular cultivar traces back to the parking lot outside of a Grateful Dead concert—a common point in many strain origin stories—in Deer Creek, IN, in 1991. Krzanowski landed an ounce of a strain called "Dogbud" that was so notably happy, giggly, and cerebral that he made sure to get a few more. One of those ounces had thirteen seeds, three of which turned out female, and from those he grew the first batch of Chem 91. That desirable strain became a hit coast-to-coast, leading to more incredible creations like OG Kush and Sour Diesel once breeders started playing with it. You might see strains labeled Chemdog or Chem 91 elsewhere, but this is the only place to get the real deal—and it happens to be a very charming, country mercantile kind of store with educated staff that's ready to answer the questions of newbies and weed nerds alike.

Open Daily

380 Dwight Street
Holyoke, MA 01040

For more locations, visit
cannaprovisions.com

THE HERITAGE CLUB

A CHARLESTOWN DISPENSARY REFERENCING THE PAST AND THE FUTURE AS THE FIRST CANNABIS SHOP IN THE STATE OWNED BY A BLACK WOMAN.

There is a bit of a speakeasy feel to The Heritage Club storefront, in the sense that you could walk right past it without knowing a vibrant, well-stocked dispensary lies within. Well, you'd probably stop to admire the mural of the red, green, and black African American flag on the exterior. First exhibited in Amsterdam, this version of the US flag was created by artist David Hammons in 1990. It flies here as a subtle art history reference that spurs a rewarding internet journey for anyone whose curiosity is piqued. In my eyes, it's a meaningful metaphor for what founder Nike John hopes to do with her dispensary: honor and reflect on the ways cannabis and Black heritage intersect. In the dispensary's name, she's also referencing her father's Caribbean heritage, plus it happens to have the initials "THC," which is a bonus.

"I knew I wanted to create a place that has style and a unique environment, a place that reflected the way weed makes you want to live in color," John said. Instead of budtenders, staff members are referred to as flight attendants. "Flight attendants help you get on and off the plane safely and provide refreshments. It feels fitting". There's a significant presence of minority-owned brands offered here, including Papi's blunts, edibles from the veteran-owned Freshly Baked, and Black Buddha flower from renowned medical cannabis activist Roz McCarthy. Adjacent to the shop is a sister space where THC hosts all kinds of community events, from infused yoga classes to comedy nights. The whole operation is a labor of love for John, who even helped paint the jewel-toned walls and tile the ornate counters herself.

Open Daily

116 Cambridge Street
Boston, MA 02129

heritageclubthc.com

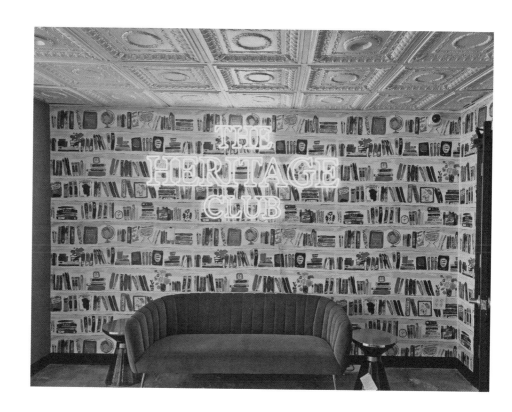

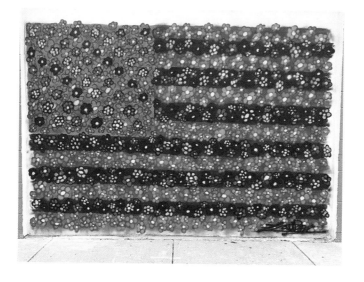

DOPE DINNERS

A HUSBAND AND WIFE'S LABOR OF LOVE, BRINGING PERSONALIZED INFUSED DINNERS TO GUESTS.

Many of the cannabis culinary experiences highlighted in this book were chosen because of the special venues and transportive environments they create. What makes Dope Dinners so special is that they bring the experience to you and execute it in the exact way you'd like. "Custom" doesn't cost extra here; it's the standard. The dinners are still transportive, don't get me wrong, but if fine dining isn't as much your crew's vibe as a big family-style brunch or next-level barbecue feast, they can work with that. You want fancy? Edgard Hunt, New England culinary expert, and Anna DeBiasi, seasoned event planner, are happy to facilitate that, too. All they need is a minimum of eight guests and a suitable venue, and then it's time to start talking menu.

The flavors often reflect the couple's Caribbean and Mediterranean heritage, influenced by whatever local New England bounty is in season. From there, they collaborate with you on any dietary restrictions, palate preferences, spice level, and THC tolerance you may have. They set the table and time the start of a curated playlist with the plating and serving of the first dish. Once the meal is served, they share some cannabis education and leave you to enjoy the night while the kitchen gets cleaned up.

One thing they won't budge on is alcohol. They don't involve alcohol in any Dope Dinners, period, which is a principle I deeply respect. I can appreciate the way alcohol can complement food and vibe, but I also wish there were more opportunities to create high-quality dining experiences that allow for *only* cannabis consumption. Alcohol has a certain impact on a high, and it doesn't take much for the combination of the two to lean toward uncomfortably intoxicated (for you and the rest of the table). That's the biggest reason they stick to signature CBD elixirs as refreshments: to cultivate joy and connection through responsible cannabis consumption.

Check out @dopedinnersbos on Instagram to attend or book your event.

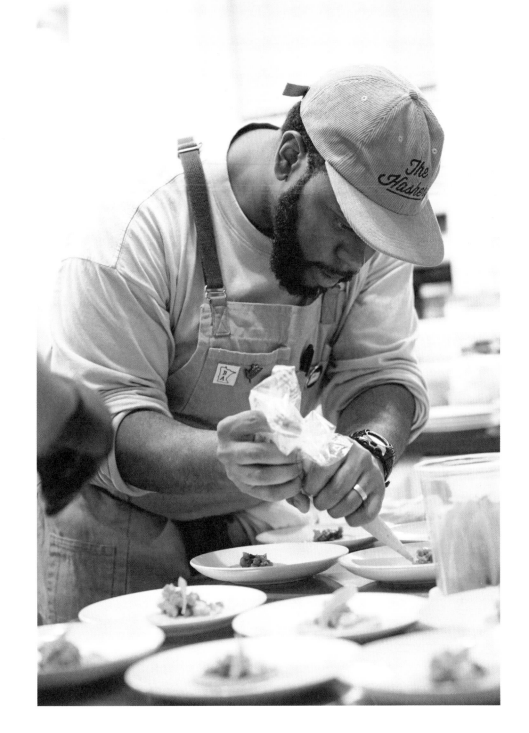

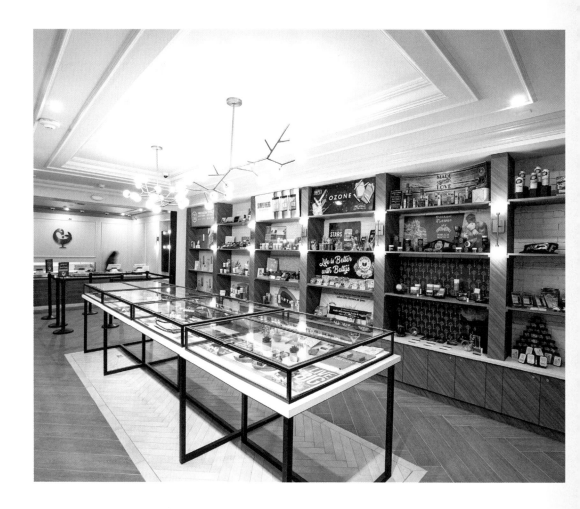

ROOTED IN

A SLEEK, COMMUNITY-ORIENTED DISPENSARY LOCATED ON ONE OF THE CITY'S COOLEST STREETS.

Founded by two local Roxbury couples, Rooted In's sophisticated space gets recommended often because of its aesthetics. It's chic and well-designed inside, offering a more upscale environment for regulars to peruse a reliably well-stocked selection of the state's finest. However, what really makes this shop special is the unique profit-sharing model innovated by the founding team.

Rooted In has fifty-five local investors, 96 percent of whom are of the BIPOC community and 50 percent of whom are women. Many are Boston residents from Roxbury, Dorchester, Mattapan, and Hyde Park. Through a shared benefits model, funds from the cannabis business are routed directly back to some of the neighborhoods that were most impacted by the War on Drugs in an effort to strengthen local communities and foster an equitable cannabis industry.

That sort of creative approach to acknowledging the negative impacts of the past and putting legal weed dollars into the communities that suffered most from its prohibition sets a meaningful example for cannabis businesses everywhere and, in my eyes, speaks volumes of the thoughtful founding team. You even see it through their design decisions. Take their logo, for example. The backward-facing bird references the Ghana sankofa bird that represents the idea that one should remember the past to make positive progress and prosperity for the future.

Open Daily

331 Newbury Street
Boston, MA 02115

rootedinroxbury.com

SACRILICIOUS

INFUSED DINNERS AND TASTING MENUS BY A MICHELIN STAR CHEF WHO BELIEVES IN THE HEALING POWER OF CANNABIS.

David Yusefzadeh is a busy guy. When I reached out to learn more about Sacrilicious, his licensed edible company Plant Jam, and his infused ice cream brand Cloud Creamery, I could hear him banging around in his commercial kitchen as we chatted, though he was quick to clarify that his executive chef Linnea Blake runs the show when it comes to the edible brands—a knee-jerk impulse to give credit where it's due that he perhaps gained from his time working in hierarchical, high-stress, fine-dining environments for much of his life.

Yusefzadeh started out as a chef at the Ritz Carlton in Atlanta, then worked in Hong Kong for a period of time at the Mandarin Oriental hotel, later running his own restaurant in his hometown of Minneapolis and helping Mario Vitaly open Eataly in Chicago. Cannabis was a part of his social life during this time, but it wasn't until he was diagnosed with Crohn's disease around 2011 that he realized just how helpful live rosin dabs were to quell his symptoms. By 2018, Yusefzadeh was able to stop taking synthetic medications altogether.

He met local event planner Sam Kanter at a cannabis event around that time, who suggested they join forces to host destination infused dinners, and Sacrilicious was born shortly after. They developed a model of five-, seven-, and nine-course tasting menus, and as the Boston cannabis scene developed, so did their schedule, from backstage VIP catering at music festivals to private events. Kanter eventually went off on her own to start an infused meal kit company, Dinner at Mary's (dinner-at-marys.com), and Yusefzadeh took the helm at Sacrilicious.

These days, he continues to work as a private chef for hire for the Boston Celtics and other non-infused gigs, but his creativity as a chef still shines brightest during these toasty dinners. He loves to experiment with the science of food, trying out fermenting miso in cannabis and curing egg yolks in weed-infused salt for a signature *amuse bouche* inspired by Dr. Seuss's green eggs and ham. When we spoke, he was giddy about an upcoming opportunity to try incorporating cannabis into the traditional cave-aging process for cheese.

To view the event schedule, visit eatsacrilicious.com

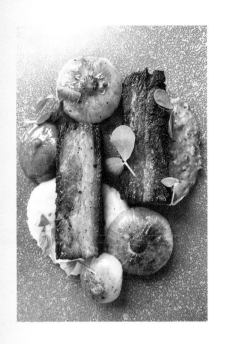

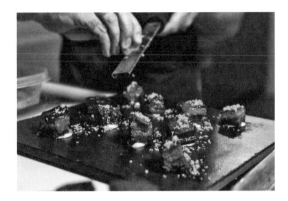

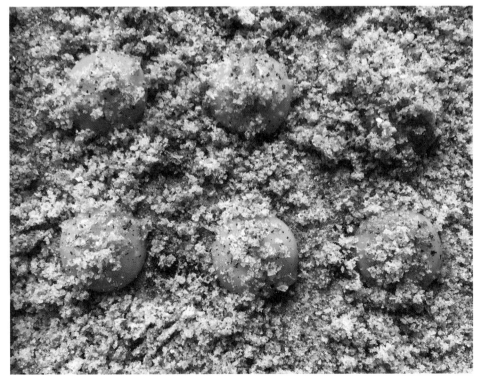

BOTERA

A POSH DISPENSARY JUST OUTSIDE THE CITY THAT TREATS FINE CANNABIS LIKE FINE JEWELRY.

As a true-blue weed lover who's never considered the word "stoner" to be an insult, I believe all shops can be great, regardless of aesthetics. Not all weed shops have to be fancy to be recommended on a top-ten list, and legitimizing cannabis as a plant doesn't require the recruitment of a design firm. That said, I believe every weed scene deserves that spot you can bring any naysayers to show them how much times have changed.

Botera, although technically outside the city, is that spot for Boston. This is where you can take your aunt who still associates cannabis with dirty, evil drugs, or where you can bring your parents when they're concerned you're throwing your career away by listing any form of cannabis work in your employment history. It's a stunning space with custom wood details and thoughtful, cozy seating areas for anyone to stop and take things in, which reminds me of a contemporary cafe in Tokyo. It's also a trustworthy shop for connoisseurs; my cannabis media colleague, Brit Smith (host of the *Different Leaf* podcast), counts this as one of her favorite shops for flower, concentrate, or topical restocks.

Open Daily

747 Centre Street
Brockton, MA 02302

boterama.com

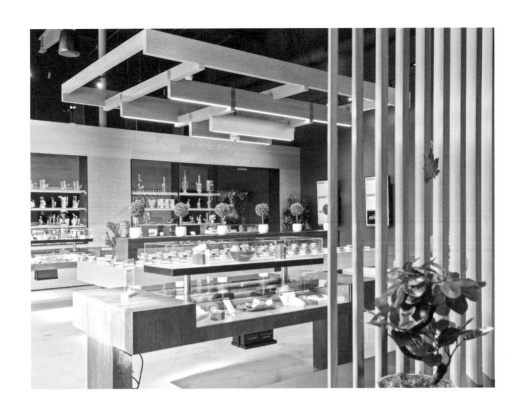

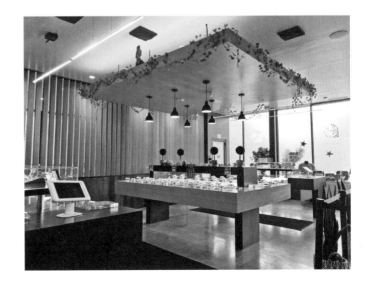

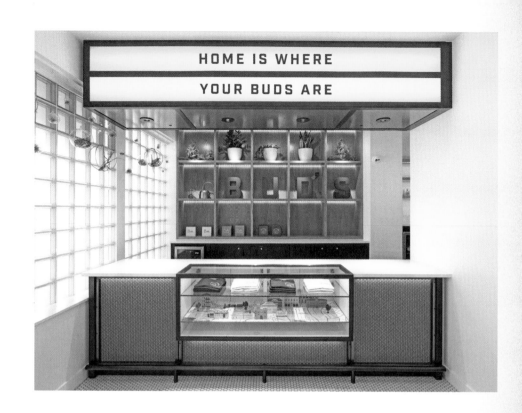

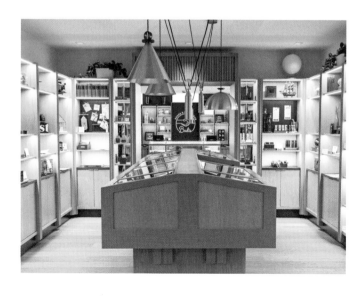

BUD'S GOODS & PROVISIONS

A LOCAL DISPENSARY CHAIN THAT HONORS THE UNIQUE VIBES OF NEW ENGLAND LOCALE AND CATERS TO THE BLUE COLLAR COMMUNITY.

You can think of the "Bud" in Bud's Goods as a friendly neighborhood dealer looking out for his hardworking homies. You might look at the very thoughtfully designed and decorated interior and question how much it's supposed to appeal to blue-collar tokers, but you know what? Everyone deserves a nice, clean, and cute neighborhood pot shop, no matter how dirty your hands get on the job.

The company operates three stores in the region: Worcester, Abington, and Watertown. Each of the locations feature custom-crafted cabinetry filled with found artifacts from yesteryear, like model ships, well-loved books, and vintage cameras. The Worcester location's layout draws inspiration from a New England diner, while Abington's design is based on a movie theater. Watertown's is modeled after "Bud's home" with a "Pantry" section for edibles and a "Library" to showcase the flower selection.

Their flower selection is the other major factor that sets this trio of stores apart. The versatile menu has a broad range of price points, from the affordable Lil' Bud's eighth of flower and Lil' Jays pre-rolls to the full-sized buds of Bud's Everyday flower and Bud's Finest flower, the latter being the top tier, primo buds sourced from legit Massachusetts farms.

Open Daily

64 W Boylston Street
Worcester, MA 01606

For more locations, visit
budsgoods.com

SUMMIT LOUNGE

A FAMILY-OWNED-AND-OPERATED LOUNGE PROVIDING MILKSHAKES, LATTES, AND CHROMECAST CONNECTIONS TO CANNABIS LOVERS IN WORCESTER.

To be clear, there aren't licenses for cannabis consumption lounges in Massachusetts. However, if consuming cannabis in private spaces is legal, then doing so—without any sales of cannabis on-site—in a private, members-only club is also allowed. That's what Kyle Moon and his family found out ahead of opening Summit Lounge in 2018.

"We operate like an Elks Lodge or a Masonic Temple," Moon explained. "The fourth and fourteenth amendments come into play here; the key here is private versus public."

If they didn't have a lawyer in the family—Moon's uncle—they wouldn't have felt confident enough to go for it. That said, after careful review, he couldn't find a reason it'd be illegal. And the Summit storefront wouldn't have been possible without the whole family pitching in, from Moon's electrician father to his brothers operating a medical grow in Maine that helped the lounge pay rent during pandemic-related closures. Together, the family owns the lounge, a restaurant, and a bowling alley, all of which are labors of love that everyone works on.

"Everything we could do ourselves, we did," Moon said.

They built a cafe inside the lounge that offers coffee, tea, milkshakes, and a variety of indulgent ice cream sundae options. Personally, it's hard to imagine a more perfect set of refreshments while sparking up some fine flower I brought from home. Local dispensaries often throw employee appreciation events here, and it's common for brands to choose this venue for their company Christmas parties. In 2022, former NFL star Ricky Williams hosted a launch party for his cannabis brand Highsman at the Lounge.

The bongs, dab rigs, and fancy Stündenglass Gravity Infusers are all cleaned daily to be like new each rental, and the ambient music is never too loud to mess up a good conversation. Social butterflies can hang at the bar, and quieter guests can pick a cozy nook and put whatever they want on the nearest TV via Chromecast devices that are attached to each.

Open Wednesday–Saturday

116 Water Street
Worcester, MA 01604

thesummitlounge.com

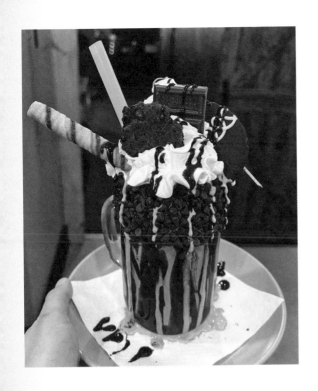

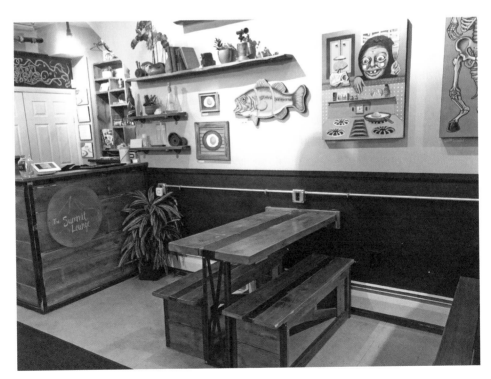

FINE FETTLE

A WELL-STOCKED, FAMILY-OWNED CHAIN OF SHOPS REACHING ACROSS STATE BORDERS AND THE MARTHA'S VINEYARD SOUND.

When Massachusetts legalized cannabis, it wasn't quite sure how to handle the island of Martha's Vineyard. Accessible only by plane or boat, the idea of thousands of pounds of weed getting transported alongside summer travelers to this vacation destination was not one that reassured local legislators. So, when Connecticut-based cannabis brand Fine Fettle wanted to branch out onto the island, they were told they didn't have that option. If they wanted to sell cannabis on Martha's Vineyard, they'd have to grow cannabis on Martha's Vineyard. Already operating three busy locations in Connecticut and one in Rowley, MA—the state's only full-service dispensary on the frequently trafficked Route 1—CEO and founder Benjamin Zachs was up for the challenge.

Today, in addition to their outdoor grow on mainland Mass., their Martha's Vineyard greenhouse and dispensary are up and popping, hosting events in the summer when the island's population quadruples. Fine Fettle, as a company, is the sort of local success I am heartened to see, proving that mom-and-pop operations doing things thoughtfully can see the same success as corporate multi-state operators with much deeper pockets.

Zachs and his team take their time finding master growers to run the multiple cultivation hubs, and, for the Martha's Vineyard grow, they even paid for an experienced Denver cultivator to relocate to the island. (Fortuitously, the grower's girlfriend was originally from Massachusetts and was happy to move back). It's clear they respect quality cannabis and what it can do, not only in regards to their business, but also in our understanding of it and the plant world at large. In fact, the company helped found a Cannabis Innovation and Research Center in the region with the hopes of connecting people who are interested in researching cannabis from all angles.

Open Daily

**116 Newburyport Turnpike
Rowley, MA 01969**

**For more locations, visit
finefettle.com**

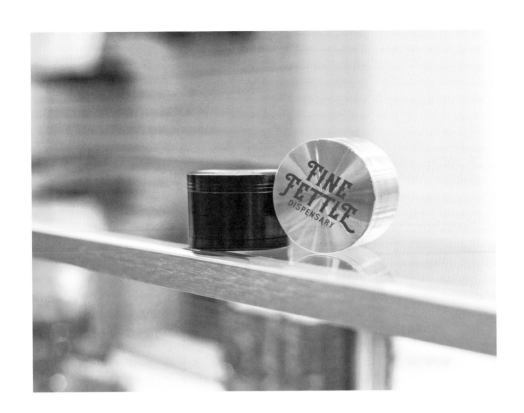

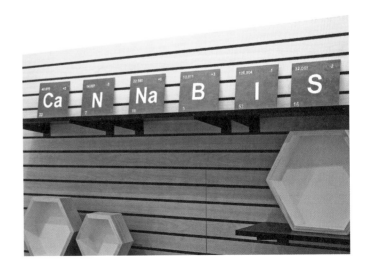

To be blunt, New Jersey legislators and law enforcement are not big fans of weed. In 2017, New Jersey arrested 34,500 people on cannabis offenses—more than any other state in the country. Even after legalization, more than 70 percent of New Jersey towns initially banned adult-use retail.

So, while the people of New Jersey are mostly down with the progression of a legal weed scene, the state isn't exactly fostering a flourishing market. Until now, the players have been mostly big medical operators with major investment backings that were able to convert to adult-use businesses. There are provisions in the state law for consumption lounges and equity licenses, but those licenses are only just now getting distributed. New companies operated by locals without big corporate ties, like delivery startup Roll Up Life, have been struggling for years to get their businesses off the ground.

I interviewed those founders about their new ventures, and sadly, they're still struggling to get through the mess of red tape and city councilors standing in their way. However, as you may have observed by now, a lack of dynamic retail spaces doesn't mean a lack of a cannabis community. There are a few key businesses laying roots down in the Garden State's slowly softening soil.

MAPLEWOOD   TRENTON   MAPLEWOOD

NEW J

LEGALIZED

Medical in 2010 (barely—it's a very strict, expensive program with a low number of patients), recreational in 2021

POSSESSION

Adults over the age of 21 can possess: one ounce cannabis flower, four grams of solid cannabis concentrates or resin (or the equivalant of four grams of concentrate), and one thousand milligrams of edibles (i.e. ten one-hundred-milligram packages).

HOME GROWS

Not legal

DELIVERY

Yes, but only to private residences (no hotels).

CONSUMPTION

Smoking is allowed on private property or at a licensed cannabis consumption space.

CITIES

Maplewood
Trenton

TRENTON

MAPLEWOOD

TRENTON

ERSEY

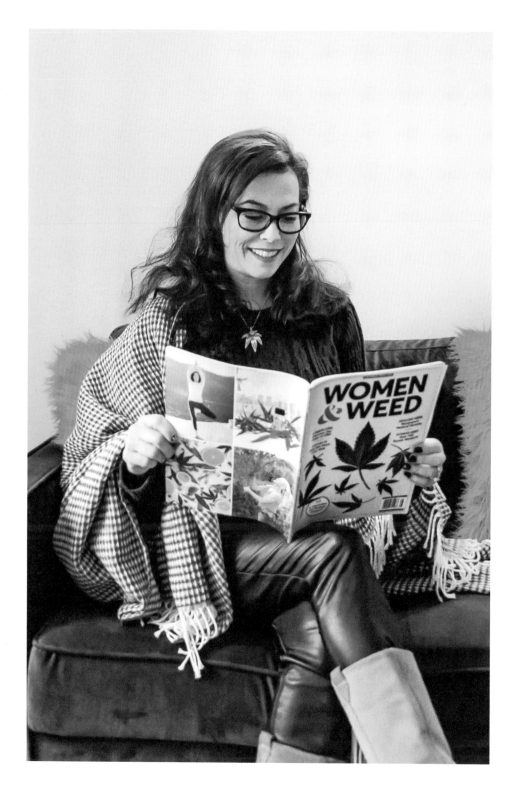

THE CANNABOSS LADY

A CHARMING CBD BOUTIQUE IN MAPLEWOOD VILLAGE WITH A LICENSED CANNABIS DISPENSARY NEXT DOOR.

When it comes to cannabis education and normalization, licensed dispensaries are only part of the equation. Many people who are still on the fence about this controversial plant aren't yet comfortable walking into a shop covered in cannabis leaf signage and pulling out their ID at the counter. What they need is a safe space somewhere in between an independent boutique and a licensed pot shop, a space that is overtly OK with cannabis, where you can openly ask questions without fear of being judged and trust that the answers will be well informed.

In a scene that has been slow to develop, where the traumas of law enforcement's actions against the community are still fresh, the CannaBoss Lady is that space—a very selfie-friendly one to boot.

Founded in 2020 by Jill Cohen, who pivoted toward the hemp and cannabis scene after discovering the positive medicinal effects for herself, the welcoming space feels like a pink-and-green-themed beauty parlor. There's ample, cushy seating for any shoppers who want to talk through how CBD works and which of the small batch, third-party tested and thoughtfully curated products might be right for them.

Cohen cares deeply about the quality of the products as well as the vendors she chooses to support, opting for fellow women and minority-owned brands whenever possible. Offerings include TribeTokes vaporizers, Bhumi edibles, and CBD-infused skincare from brands like Potency No. 710, whose gold face serum Cohen describes as a "fountain of youth." Cohen also coordinates events and meetups in her space and around town, bringing together entrepreneurs and curious consumers for networking brunches and helpful workshops, like CBD and Menopause 101.

Open Tuesday–Sunday

9 Highland Place
Maplewood, NJ 07040

thecannabosslady.com

THE APOTHECARIUM

A CALIFORNIA-GROWN DISPENSARY CHAIN THAT'S QUICKLY EARNED A SPOT IN LOCAL CONNOISSEUR'S HEARTS.

Born in the Bay Area, the Apothecarium served as one of the very first instances of high-end design in cannabis dispensaries. Rather than catering to the youngest, most stoned customers, co-founder Ryan Hudson aimed to create a space that his grandmother would feel comfortable visiting, a place that looked and felt so nice that it wouldn't invite judgment or make her self-conscious when walking inside, a mature ambiance that didn't feel too stuffy.

He succeeded, as their flagship location in the Castro District of San Francisco was once named the best-designed dispensary in the country by *Architectural Digest*. The same modern farmhouse-styled interior can be found at the three New Jersey locations of the Apothecarium, where stately marble countertops are illuminated by chic lighting fixtures.

Aside from a trusted curation of consumable goods, this is a great spot to shop for interesting smokeware. You'll find high-design pieces so cool you'll want to leave it out on your coffee table, plus you'll be happy to know there's always a knowledgeable budtender there to help you figure out the right handheld flower vape for your needs.

Open Daily

**1865 Springfield Avenue
Maplewood, NJ 07040**

**For more locations, visit
apothecarium.com**

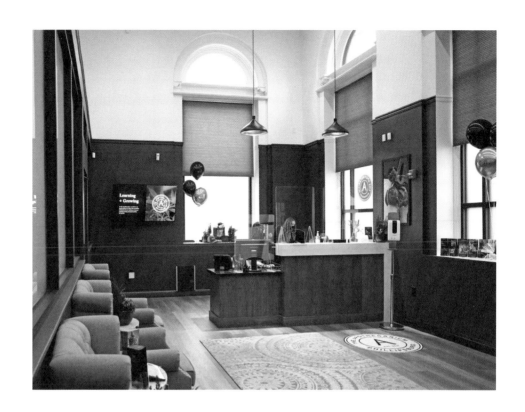

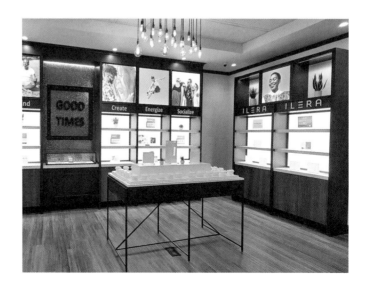

SIMPLY PURE TRENTON

THE FIRST EAST COAST OUTPOST OF THE RENOWNED COLORADO DISPENSARY, OPERATED BY RENOWNED SOCIAL JUSTICE ADVOCATES.

Related to the Simply Pure founded by Wanda James (see p. 134) in Denver, CO, this Simply Pure offers the same educated and experienced service with a dose of real New Jersey flavor. James is less interested in expanding her empire as she is widening the door for more Black cannabis entrepreneurs to follow in her footsteps and find success in their home state, tapping individuals with a passion for cannabis advocacy to lead her new out-of-state locations.

Simply Pure Trenton is led by noted social equity advocate and Trenton native Tahir Johnson, who's been involved with influential organizations like the Marijuana Policy Project, the US Cannabis Council, and the National Cannabis Industry Association. Johnson also dealt with a cannabis-related arrest in his youth, making him someone who now gets to rewrite his relationship with the plant as a legal, leading entrepreneur in his hometown. While James maintains some conversation with the look and feel of the place, she's empowered the local managers to customize the store environment to fit the communities they serve. It's about being a *neighborhood* shop, not a Colorado franchise. This is Johnson's show, and James is just happy to provide the platform to give Trenton the trustworthy dispensary they deserve.

Open Daily

1531 N Olden Avenue
Ewing Township, NJ 08638

For more locations, visit
simplypuretrenton.com

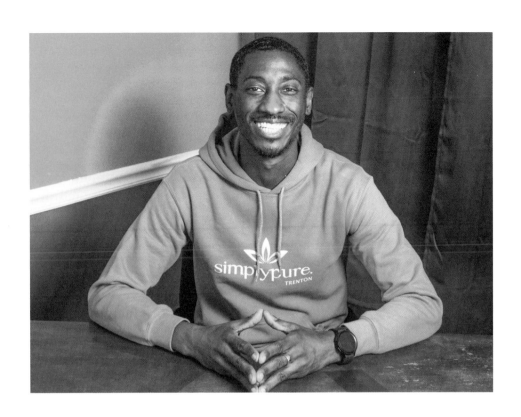

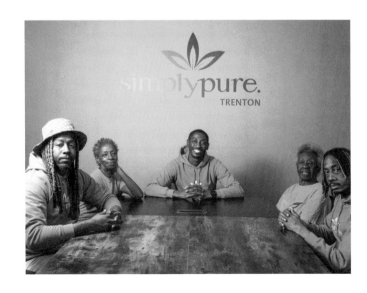

It isn't possible to tell the story of modern cannabis without a stop in New York City. From jazz musicians' legendary reefer-fueled riffs to the musings of Beat authors and the cloudy crowds surrounding the Woodstock festival stage in Bethel, New York, as Jimi Hendrix strummed a psychedelic rendition of the National Anthem—culturally, cannabis has always had a home here. It was also on these streets where harmful stop-and-frisk policing was born in the 1990s, devastating Black and Latino communities and making the city the cannabis arrest capital of America.

Then, just like that, cannabis became more legal here than nearly anywhere else. I still can't believe you can smoke anywhere cigarettes are allowed. New York's legalization laws went further than any state that came before them in an attempt to right some of the wrongs committed in the name of the War on Drugs, namely giving priority to applicants for dispensary licenses who were legacy New Yorkers from communities most impacted by cannabis prohibition and those with past cannabis-related charges. The New York Police Department immediately directed cops to adapt their stance to reflect legalization, and an unprecedented boom of a gray cannabis market emerged in the waiting time for dispensaries to get approved through this more nuanced—and subsequently, more complicated and litigious—licensing process.

While I hope you make it to a neighborhood bodega for a breakfast sandwich, I'd wait until you get inside of a licensed dispensary to pick up your buds. It won't be as convenient as any of the illicit weed trucks you might pass along the way, but I promise the trustworthy, lab-tested quality of the products are worth it.

NEW

LEGALIZED

Medical in 2014,
recreational in 2021

POSSESSION

Adults over the age of
21 can possess: three
ounces of cannabis
flower and twenty-four
grams of concentrate
or edibles

HOME GROWS

For now, no. Only medical
patients and caregivers
can grow plants at home.

 DELIVERY

Yes, but only to private
residences (no hotels).

CONSUMPTION

Adults may smoke or
vape cannabis wherever
smoking tobacco is
allowed, with a few
exceptions. That's right;
it's legal right out on
the street.

 CITIES

New York City

NEW YORK CITY   NEW YORK CITY   NEW YOR

YORK

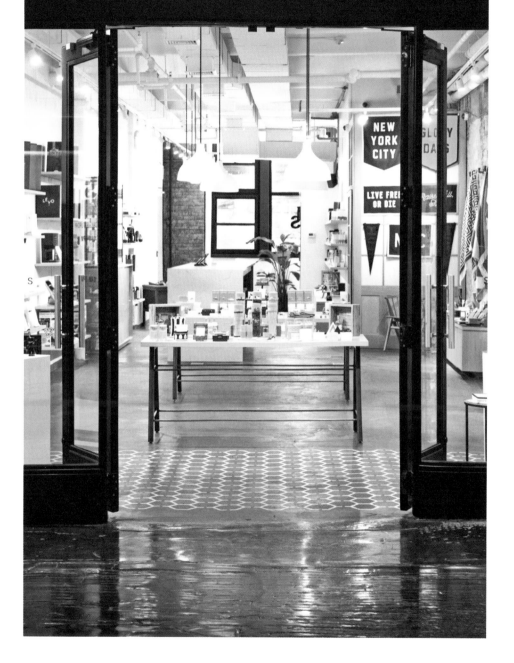

HIGHER STANDARDS

A HIGH-CLASS SPIN ON THE CLASSIC ACCESSORY-FILLED HEAD SHOP NESTLED IN CHELSEA MARKET.

There are few experiences as shockingly tragic as the moment you break your bong or the moment you realize you've run out of rolling papers. All of a sudden, the fun that was about to be had is no more—not until you get yourself to a smoke shop, or head shop, however you refer to a convenience store that sells Zig Zag rolling papers and bongs called "water pipes for tobacco."

The average smoke shop is, well, average, selling bare necessities from random mass manufacturers. Higher Standards is truly a luxury version of that, selling well-curated accessories for consuming cannabis as well as modern cannabis-reverent art and decor to complete your contemporary stoner home. I appreciate their straightforward house line of practical glass smoking pieces and their fantastic assortment of cleaning materials designed to effectively clean those uncommon shapes (something so hard to do and something we all should be doing more regularly).

You can peruse chic ashtrays and storage containers, high-tech grinders, and smoke-disguising candles, plus Higher Standards' collabs like Jonathan Adler coasters and well-made, smell-proof goods by Revelry—the backpack of which I use every time I leave the house with anything fragrant.

Located in Chelsea Market, a maze of restaurants and shops in New York City's Meatpacking District, the gallery-like space is a great place to reintroduce someone to cannabis, particularly if they hold on to stigma around the sketchiness or questionable nature of this plant. One look at the polished pieces made for the sole purpose of accompanying and complementing cannabis, set in this sophisticated space in the mix of other cool boutiques and eateries, and it's hard to remember what the prohibitive fuss was all about.

Open Daily

75 9th Avenue
New York, NY 10011

higherstandards.com

HOUSING WORKS CANNABIS CO.

NEW YORK CITY'S FIRST LEGAL DISPENSARY LED BY ONE OF THE CITY'S MOST BELOVED NONPROFITS.

Located in Manhattan, Housing Works Cannabis Co. is something of our cannabis activist foremothers' dreams. The dispensary is operated by Housing Works, an established city nonprofit known for its decades of work in AIDS rights and affordable housing advocacy. All proceeds from Housing Works Cannabis Co. support the nonprofit side, just like the organization's long-beloved resale shops and book store in Soho.

It's special that these were the first people earning income from legal cannabis sales in the state, not only because of their work, but because, as an organization, Housing Works has long held a nuanced, nonpunitive approach to drug use in their clientele. They've walked the walk for a long time, and now they're doing it with legal cannabis.

Overall, the space is welcoming and uplifting, adorned with posters reading "Make Love, Not Drug War." The counters and displays are illuminated with a pastel color spectrum, mirroring the way it feels to exhale cannabis and feel the weight start to lift from your shoulders. For that rainbow-hued haze of relief, there's regeneratively grown flower from Florist Farms out of Cortland, NY—in bud, pre-roll, or vape form—and edibles from interesting brands like Ayrloom, a family-run company that's operated an apple farm in Lafayette, NY, for over a hundred years.

Open Daily

**750 Broadway
New York, NY 10003**

hwcannabis.co

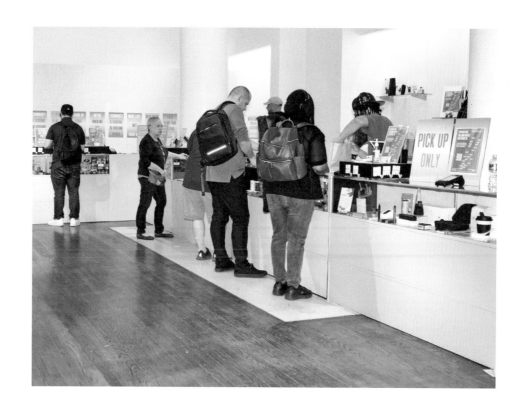

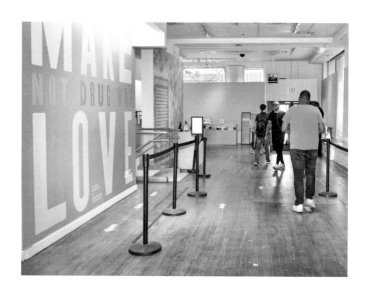

VIC STYLES, CANNABIS ADVOCATE AND FOUNDER OF BLACK GIRLS SMOKE

blackgirlssmoke.com

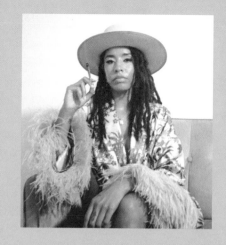

When Vic Styles landed in Los Angeles in 2010, she was set on a rich, rewarding career in the fashion industry. She ran a blog about her experiences while working as a wardrobe stylist— around the same time a new app called Instagram was resonating with millennials everywhere. She started an Instagram account to accompany her blog, sharing curated snippets of the fashion realm and incorporating plant medicine practices passed down from her herbalist mother. She quickly found herself at the forefront of the wellness influencer game, receiving products and brands deals to document her experiences.

Eventually she launched the cannabis brand Good Day Flor and Black Girls Smoke, a community dedicated to showing the world that Black women can be entrepreneurs, moms, educated, classy, "grown AF," *and* smoke. Members of the Black Girls Smoke community get access to a monthly book club, active job board, wellness workshops, industry experts, and resources for starting a cannabis-related business. I connected with Styles over the phone to learn more about Black Girls Smoke and the still-establishing legal weed rhythms of the city that never sleeps.

HOW DID BLACK GIRLS SMOKE COME ABOUT?

When I moved to NYC in 2019, I didn't have many friends. I also had a manager for the first time, who was like, "You want big brand partnerships? You can't be smoking online." So, I was like, "OK, I'll start a separate Instagram account." That was the birth of Black Girls Smoke. No one else was talking to Black women who enjoyed cannabis at the time, so it blew up. I had no plans or vision for it; it was the community that started shaping it into what it's become. They wanted to connect, so when 4/20 rolled around [the unofficial but widely celebrated holiday for weed], we held a virtual party with poet Jasmine Mans—creator of the Buy Weed From Women campaign—and music artist Lizzy Jeff, aka Rap Priestess. This was 2020, when the COVID-19 pandemic was happening, and we only had one thousand followers at the time.

We did our first in-person experience in August 2020 called Puff in the Park. About ten to twenty people showed up, and everyone was like twenty feet apart, but we got to smoke together and connect in person, safely. The following August, there were over three thousand RSVPs to the second installment of Puff in the Park.

WHAT WAS IT LIKE TO LEAVE THE WEST COAST'S WEED SCENE FOR NEW YORK'S?

It was a bit of a culture shock to leave Los Angeles, where I could order nice weed via Eaze, and then land in New York and go back to getting weed from guys I don't know. Once the state legalized, everybody decided to start selling weed. All of a sudden my corner bodega went from selling just papers and lighters to selling flower. There's still so much gray area stuff. I think people have transitioned to buying vapes and edibles in licensed dispensaries faster because you want to trust that it's safe and that it is what it says it is. But when you can see and smell bodega flower, it's easy to feel like it looks safe.

HOW WOULD YOU DESCRIBE NEW YORK CANNABIS CULTURE?

If you take out the cannabis, Los Angeles culture can be a little superficial, putting visual appeal and aesthetics first. In New York, there's a bit more of a culture and community feel, especially where I am in Brooklyn. There's more Blackness. Regardless of cannabis, I hope New York becomes the new Amsterdam. There are already millions of tourists arriving weekly. I hope some of those become niche tourists that are just here for the weed.

My grandma always says, "How you do one thing is how you do everything," and I imagine New York cannabis in that way. The way there are so many subcultures here—in fashion, nightlife, music, etc.—I'm ready for art girl weed, New York Fashion Week weed, Bronx boys weed, etc. I believe New York can really help weed become a lifestyle element and not a drug.

MOST SOCIAL MEDIA PLATFORMS ARE INCREASINGLY HOSTILE TO BRANDS THAT POST ABOUT CANNABIS AND HEMP. PERHAPS IT'LL CHANGE IF AND WHEN FEDERAL LEGALIZATION HAPPENS, PERHAPS NOT. DOES THAT WORRY YOU FOR BLACK GIRLS SMOKE'S SUSTAINABILITY?

I think we have to adapt. Look at how people adapted from TV commercials to podcast platforms and digital ads. Social media is the number one source of marketing, so we have to figure out how to survive on these platforms. We have to think outside of the box. Maybe you can't show a joint being smoked, but you can show munchie snacks, for example. Now that I'm a CEO, I'm interested in how we adapt, in seeing how media and storytelling evolve in general. I am thinking bigger than Instagram or TikTok; we envision a media world of BGS not unlike *ESSENCE*.

TONIC

A HEMP-TURNED-CANNABIS BRAND THAT ADVOCATES FOR THE PLANT, THE PEOPLE, AND TRANSPARENCY.

As someone who started in the medical cannabis space, I was completely freaked out when the hemp CBD craze emerged. To this day, there's no head of the hemp world. That's why, for many years, when someone asked for a reliable CBD topical for sore muscles or a tincture for mental calm, I recommended TONIC. I interviewed the founder, Long Island native Brittany Carbone, for an article that centered around the tours she'd hosted at her hemp farm in 2018, and the more we talked, the more I was impressed.

Carbone and her husband grew and harvested their own hemp, processed the plant material themselves, and formulated their own products. Carbone was among the only independent CBD brands growing their own hemp in 2017, and she was also an early face at cannabis-related events in general, helping build a new cannabis community of

people looking to get into the legal cannabis or hemp game.

In addition to inviting tours out to the farm, Carbone is passionate about empowering people to make the most of their newfound right to grow cannabis at home and connecting good people, like when she helped Housing Works, New York's first legal shop, get in touch with trusted, licensed brands when they were frantically filling shelves for launch. Now, TONIC has a THC line of vapes, gummies, and pre-rolls stocked in New York dispensaries in addition to their hemp CBD offerings, which is a damn good thing because while I am a fan of their gummies, their CBD face oil remains my skin's favorite weed-related product.

For list of stockists, visit tonicvibes.com

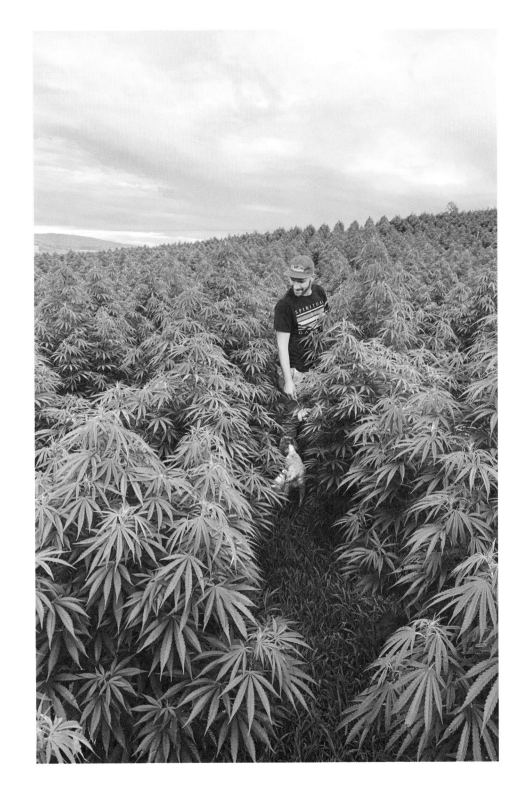

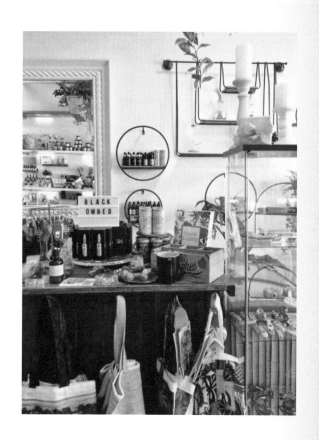

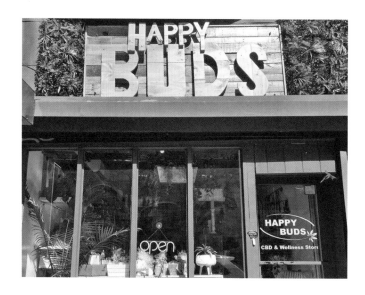

HAPPY BUDS

A BROOKLYN HEMP BOUTIQUE HOSTING FUN EVENTS AND STOCKING MOST OF THE BEST CBD BRANDS FROM ACROSS THE COUNTRY.

All kinds of stores sell CBD these days—bougie grocery stores, convenience stores, and many vintage shops and hair salons—but, in all of these instances, CBD is rarely the star of the show. Alternatively, Happy Buds celebrates CBD, hemp, and herbal alternatives by highlighting the craft and caring makers of these products, not unlike a specialty wine shop. This makes sense, as Happy Buds is run by the same people behind Happy Cork, a Brooklyn wine store that became a fast hit with their well-curated offerings reflecting diverse vintners.

Sunshine and Remo Foss took the same approach with Happy Buds, thoughtfully sourcing products made by many minority- and women-owned brands, like tinctures and CBD capsules from Plant People, skin-soothing CBD oils by Earth's Dew, and various forms of balms and creams by Not Pot. They were early stockists of Zero Two Four, a Brooklyn-based company making candles that are scientifically formulated to eliminate the smell of torched cannabis, and one of the few places around stocking a bunch of Burning Love's very cute smoking accessories, like ashtrays and storage containers decorated with whimsical shrooms and retro blooms. Plenty of people find themselves inside the cozy, botanical space for other reasons than just a resupply, though, as they often resituate the upcycled furnishings to make room for intimate cannabis-centric gatherings and dinners.

Open Daily

**225 Malcolm X Boulevard
Brooklyn, NY 11221**

happybudsbk.com

HIGHER DINING

A SISTER-OPERATED INFUSED CATERING AND EVENT COMPANY CREATING INTIMATE EXPERIENCES WITH DOMINICANA FLAIR.

Growing up in a female-dominated, Dominican family, Roshelly and Shanelly Pena were given strong examples of badass women through their mother and grandmother. However, their father—a lifelong student of cannabis—was the one who really inspired the idea for Higher Dining. The pair of sisters had found their way to enjoying cannabis at different points in their youth, but once they aligned on their floral belief systems, it was hard to ignore what powerful connections both food and cannabis can foster. Good food and good cannabis both bring people together, and they wanted to do the same in a stylish, aesthetic way.

In 2017, they hosted their first Higher Dining event, a four-course meal topped with a traditional Dominican tres leche cake, hosted in their mom's backyard with styled place settings and lots of flower for guests to smoke as they pleased. When the COVID-19 pandemic hit, they started offering infused plate dinners for delivery in the Bronx, routinely selling out as New Yorkers sought out ways to celebrate special occasions while the city was shut down.

Higher Dining continues to evolve as the Pena sisters' lives and families grow, adding cooking classes, private catered events, and seasonal, consumption-friendly yoga sessions to their services. They still call up their parents for tips on tweaking family recipes, bouncing ideas off of their family when working ancestral ingredients into modern menus. One themed spread for a past Eastern-inspired dinner shows their creativity and sense of adventure with their dishes: blazed shrimp with spicy chili, pot slaw, trippy Brussels, high short ribs, smacked coconut rice, and Filipino halo-halo for dessert. For a past Galentine's Day event, they baked a handful of simple white cakes and provided materials for an intimate cake decorating class. If you've got an occasion or just a craving to connect with other people who enjoy cannabis and good food in New York, the Pena sisters got you.

For event schedule, visit higherdining.com

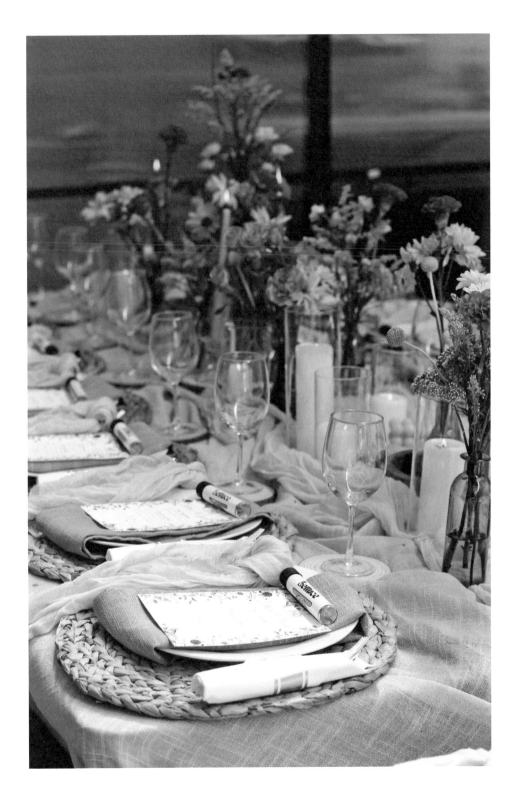

HEMP LAB NYC

A PAIR OF CBD SHOPS BY STONERS, FOR STONERS, WITH VINTAGE READS AND THREADS ON HAND.

Hemp Lab NYC started with the smoke-filled friendship of New York natives Stephanie Diaz and Manos Lupassakis, which stretches back to their high school days. The pair later ran multiple cannabis gardens within Washington state's medical system, immersing themselves in growing, processing, and better understanding this plant before making their way back to New York City five years later. They wanted to create space that would allow for others to learn about and celebrate the plant together, and once they found the Bushwick location, sitting on top of underground jazz club Wilson Live, they knew they had something.

Hemp Lab NYC opened in 2018, and their Greenpoint location followed a couple of years later, featuring a consumption-friendly private patio that hosts all kinds of events and gatherings. People hang out there on laptops as much as they come by to pick up vetted CBD lotions and potions. Events range from "Pipe Craft" series, during which attendees get to make functional ceramic smoking vessels, to "Indigo 101," where people learn about the ancient art of *shibori* and upcycling using plant dyes. Both locations carry a curated selection of vintage goods, including clothing, deadstock rolling papers, and vintage cannabis magazines and accessories.

Open Daily

**637 Wilson Avenue, BRM 2
Brooklyn, NY 11207**

**For more locations, visit
hemplabnyc.com**

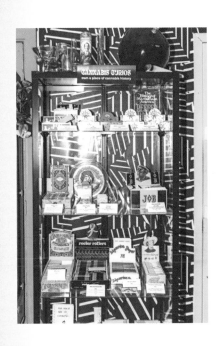

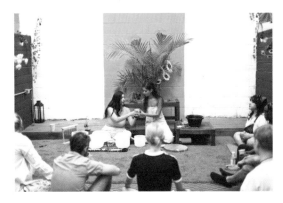

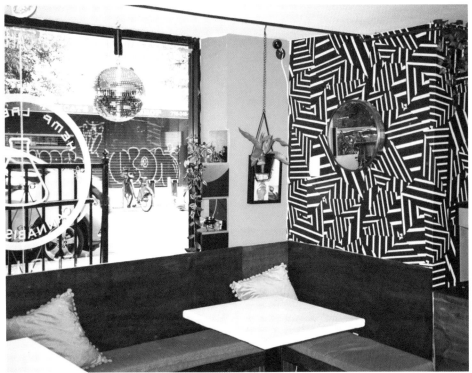

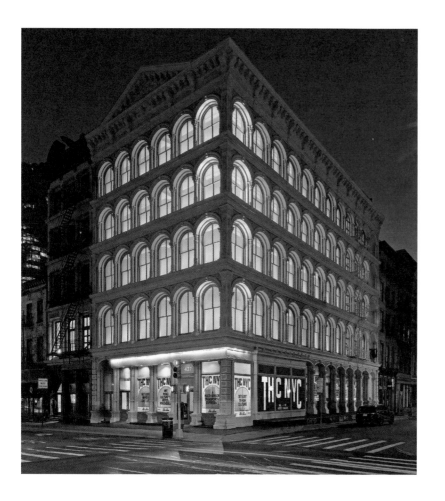

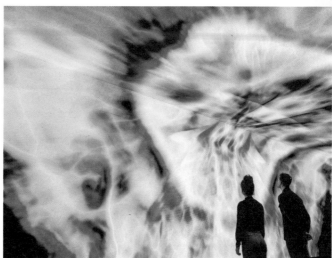

THE HOUSE OF CANNABIS

A FIVE-STORY INTERACTIVE MUSEUM AND GALLERY DEDICATED TO EVERY ASPECT OF CANNABIS CULTURE.

The House of Cannabis—aka THCNYC—is a sort of new-age cultural institution centered around cannabis. Occupying an impressive historic cast-iron building on Broadway, the museum is home to over ten immersive exhibits that celebrate and investigate the many facets of our relationship with this magical plant.

The journey starts on the fourth floor with a green-hued, multimedia experience that walks guests through some of the biggest moments in the long, several-thousand-year history of cannabis, then leads them to The Euphorium, a music-inspired exhibit featuring a giant turntable big enough for you and a friend or two to lay out on while enjoying a light and music show created by famed lighting designer Michael Potvin of Nitemind.

Continuing down the floors and exhibits, you can expect curations of short films; spoken word; gallery spaces showing various artists and designers' interpretations of cannabis-related subcultures; a real, living mini cannabis grow; an olfactory-focused, aromatic exhibit made with terpenes; and a lot more. There's also a munchy-minded café, private work and lounge areas if inspiration strikes (it likely will), and—like any respected cultural institution—a gift shop.

Open Wednesday–Sunday

427 Broadway
New York, NY 10013

thcnyc.com

UNION SQUARE TRAVEL AGENCY

A NONPROFIT-OPERATED DISPENSARY HELPING THE HOUSELESS AND FORMERLY INCARCERATED FIND PERMANENT HOUSING.

One of the first legal dispensaries to open its doors in New York City, Union Square Travel Agency is another instance of a purpose-driven nonprofit earning a coveted cannabis dispensary license. More than half of all proceeds from the shop go to The Doe Fund, an organization leading the charge against homelessness and recidivism by providing paid employment, transitional and permanent housing, and support services to people who have experienced homelessness and incarceration.

This doesn't feel like the average not-for-profit environment, though; Union Square Travel Agency is a transportive, upscale space with dramatic, floor-to-ceiling red tassels around the entrance and white tassel art dangling from above like chandeliers in their violet-hued showroom.

In addition to an ever-expanding assortment of flower, edibles, and vape options, you can find stylish ceramic one-hitter pipes from House of Puff, *Broccoli* magazines that, depending on the issue, may include an article from yours truly, and marble ashtrays from Her Highness. In addition to the selfie-ready aesthetics and positive impact of dollars spent here, there's another major, less-direct perk: Union Square Travel Agency happens to be located a block away from the storied, sprawling, near century-old Strand bookstore.

Open Daily

62 E 13th Street
New York, NY 10003

unionsquaretravelagency.com

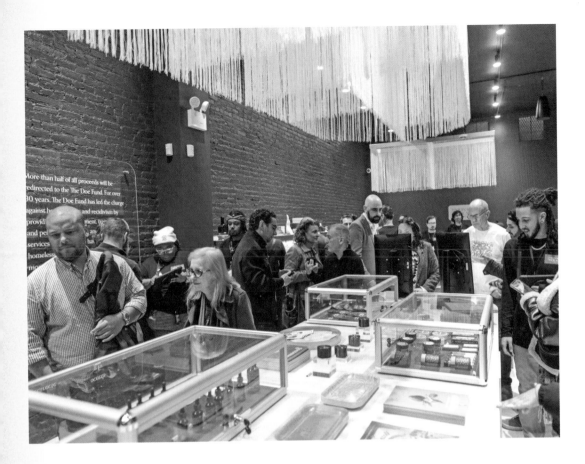

BEND & BLAZE YOGA

CANNABIS-FRIENDLY YOGA SESSIONS HELD IN COOL VENUES ACROSS THE CITY.

Yoga is a logical complement to cannabis, and the many weed yoga activities across the country reflect the enduring allure of heightening your awareness of your body and quieting your mind with a little THC before class. However, the challenge of finding landlords that welcome a regular hotbox of cannabis smoke in their spaces also endures. Running a successful cannabis yoga series that lasts longer than a year or so requires creativity and resourcefulness, a combination demonstrated beautifully by Bend & Blaze Yoga, a cannabis consumption-friendly yoga class founded by Amanda Hitz with off-shoots in Colorado and Missouri.

Hitz leads multiple classes weekly in New York City, rotating between cannabis-friendly spaces like Bushwick artist studios, The Hussle Lab, and the multi-use space of Work 'n' Roll in Chelsea. While each class has its own vibe from the energy of that neighborhood, every Bend & Blaze class features the same modifiable routines that work for beginners and advanced yogis, as well as Hitz' patient guidance and eclectic hip-hop/psychedelic/ folk playlists. Hitz has been teaching cannabis-infused classes for several years now, so she's able to react and adjust when she notices people requiring a slower or faster pace, and she prides herself on teaching to the whole room, keeping every class fresh for the longtime Blazers.

Guests can bring their own cannabis and mat, and the first twenty minutes of class serve as time to consume together and set the tone. If they're in need of a tune-up later, folks are welcome to spark up at any time throughout.

For class schedule, visit bendandblaze.yoga

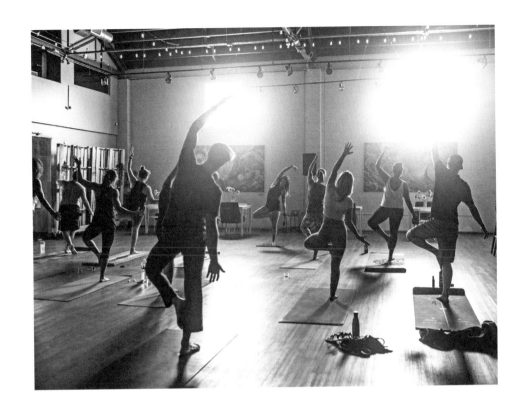

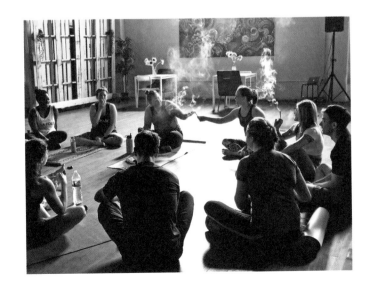

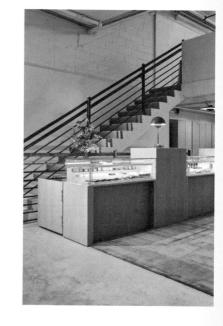

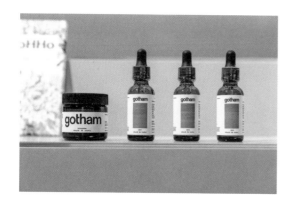

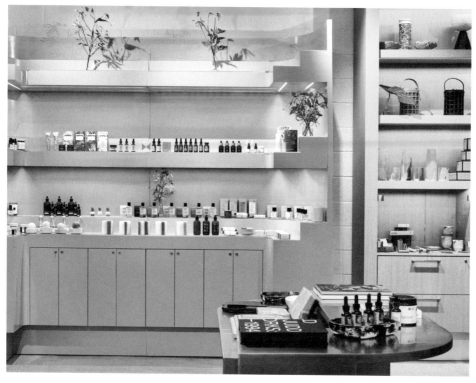

GOTHAM

AN ARTFULLY CURATED DISPENSARY MEETS A CANNABIS CONCEPT STORE ON THE BOWERY.

Honesty time: When Gotham founder Joanne Wilson's assistant reached out to me to be a guest on Wilson's *Gotham Gal* podcast, I did not know who she was. However, it didn't take longer than a couple minutes into our conversation for me to realize how much thought she'd put into the cannabis space, and from there, a fun, free-flowing conversation with a badass entrepreneur ensued. It wasn't until the end of our long chat about my path in cannabis and the state of weed culture and business that she made a small mention of a dispensary she would be opening in the coming months. I made a mental note of it, and that was that.

Fast-forward to April 2023 and not only did I see imagery of Gotham-branded flower jars decorated with the works of artists like Mark Rothko and Jeff Koons, I heard about Gotham getting the exclusive launch of Rose New York (see p. 24) in the form of their signature edible Delights, in a flavor made in collaboration with David Zilber of globally acclaimed restaurant Noma. They also carry smokables and coveted wearables by Edie Parker, a house CBD line and House of Puff accessories, among much more.

Housed in a two-story retail and gallery space, Wilson envisioned a cannabis-infused spin on concept stores like the late Colette boutique in Paris, highlighting art, fashion, and lifestyle brands as sincerely as they present premium, curated cannabis offerings. There is a permanent installation by NYC-based multimedia artist Molly Lowe and rotating exhibits that feature different NYC creators throughout the year.

Gotham operates in partnership with STRIVE, a nonprofit organization based in East Harlem that provides pathways to substantial careers for those who face societal barriers to economic empowerment, including those impacted by the justice system and those who were formerly incarcerated for cannabis. I have nothing but respect for Wilson and her team as they work to progress cannabis culture through aesthetics and social justice.

Open Daily

3 East 3rd Street
New York, NY 10003

gotham.nyc

The petite size of Vermont has proved to be its best asset when it comes to legal weed. For one, there's a long-established value for local, craft agriculture, and no one's too far from a farm. The creativity of the craft beer scene has ballooned, bringing tourists seeking farm-to-table fare on their plates and in their bongs. Legislators kept local cultivators in mind when sussing out regulations, including elements to the laws that gave a leg up to smaller businesses and attempted to slow down multistate operators with deep pockets via limits on dispensary chains. There's also a small enough number of cultivators that a novel degree of trust exists with legislators, who are totally cool with growers housing their licensed grow in their backyard. That means that instead of the hundreds of thousands of dollars typically required to become a licensed grower—millions, in many states—people from all kinds of economic backgrounds are able to get a foot in the door. Again, because of the size, most of the cultivators in Vermont are just that—passionate home growers who've grown really great weed at home for years.

That's all enough for this flower consumer to start tracking flights to the Green Mountain State, but it actually gets better. This is the only state in the country where the laws allow one to bring a mason jar from home for refills. You get to smell the flower straight from the jar, see it weighed out deli-style, and never have to use those silly plastic drams required across the West Coast and other states. I suppose it shouldn't come as a shock that the cannabis community from this haven of natural, mountainous beauty—and maple syrup—is in tune with the flora all around them, but, until cannabis is federally legalized, it remains a rare luxury to connect with local cannabis farmers so directly.

BURLINGTON RUTLAND BURLINGTON

VERM

LEGALIZED

Medical in 2004,
recreational in 2018

POSSESSION

Adults over the age of
21 can possess: up to
one ounce of cannabis
flower or no more than
five grams of concentrate
or concentrates in
edible form

HOME GROWS

Adults can grow two
mature cannabis
plants or four immature
cannabis plants.

DELIVERY

Not legal

CONSUMPTION

Smoking is allowed on
private property or in
licensed consumption
spaces.

CITIES

Burlington
Rutland

RUTLAND   BURLINGTON   RUTLAND

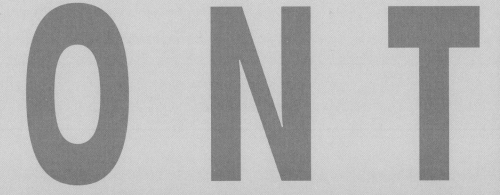

GRASS QUEEN

A BOUTIQUE-STYLED DISPENSARY CREATED BY WOMEN FOR WOMEN—AND ANYONE NOT AT HOME IN SHOPS BUILT FOR BROS.

Grass Queen is a women-owned, majority queer-owned cannabis company founded by Jahala Dudley, a seventh generation Vermonter who had yet to feel truly comfortable in an adult-use dispensary.

"I was a licensed grower in Denver, had a short stint with a Vermont medical dispensary, and I am also a cut flower farmer," Dudley said. "One of the big ideas behind Grass Queen was to escape the bro culture that's so prominent in the legal marketplace."

She set out to accomplish this in both the safe, female-friendly ambiance at Grass Queen and the products on its shelves, supporting marginalized growers and makers in the community whenever possible. Through the hot pink door and past the Pride flag, you'll find high-quality CBD and THC topicals by Vermont Organic Solutions; fantastic, regeneratively grown flower from Full Circle

Farms; and frozen, "take-and-bake" style edibles by Fog Valley Farm—all operated by women. The space features fun accessories and post-sesh reading materials, and the custom resin counter is inlaid with real cut flowers from Dudley's farm. She sought out vintage posters from the Reefer Madness era to frame for the shop's walls, especially the ones that make women the center of this plant's threatening presence, which Dudley finds equal parts hilarious and gross. They're a reminder of both the old stereotypes and the dominating male gaze that have held back cannabis culture for far too long.

Open Daily

71 S Union Street
Burlington, VT 05401

grassqueenvt.com

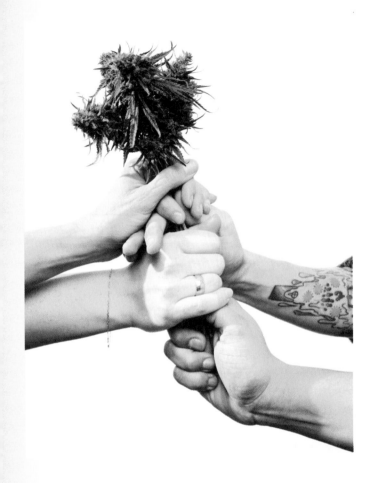
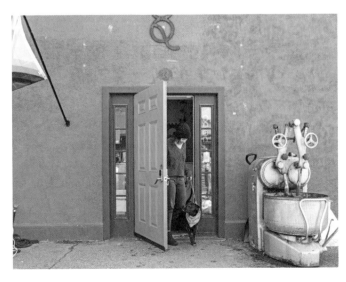

MAGIC MANN

A TRUSTED, TRUE BLUE WOMAN-OWNED SHOP WITH A MISSION TO SUPPORT A NATIVE PRESENCE IN CANNABIS.

Named after owner, founder, and widely respected woman in weed, Meredith Mann, this sweet little shop comes highly recommended by connoisseurs and newbies alike. Mann was a grower and patient in the state's medical program prior to opening the shop in 2019 with her husband and cultivation partner of twenty-one years.

The pair adhere to extremely high standards for anything that touches their shelves, from heavy-hitting, glittering buds and healing tinctures to an edible array of cautiously vetted gummies, chocolates, and low-dose beverages. They don't stock anything without a test result they didn't carefully review, and nothing is ever grown with pesticides or additives. That includes the assortment of Like a DIY CBD bath salt stations, where you can select your own flowers and essential oils for a custom-blend hemp skincare and non-infused refreshments like a locally made honey mead.

If you don't know what you want, no worries; the team is helpful and patient, and often includes Meredith herself. For a shop that's only been open for a few years, they've already had a significant impact on the community. By 2023, their internal nonprofit, the Global Indigenous Fund, raised $18,000 for a Global Indigenous Grant to be awarded to an Indigenous person or a multigenerational Vermonter seeking a start in the cannabis industry.

Open Daily

21 Essex Way, Suite 216
Essex Junction, VT 05452

magicmann.com

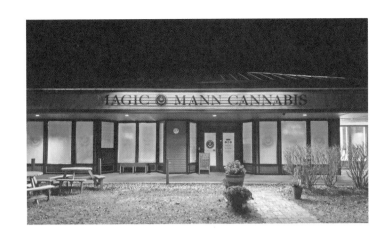

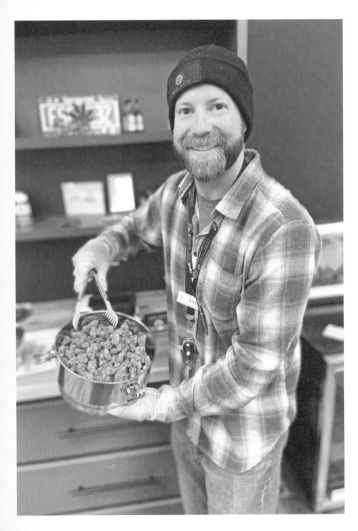

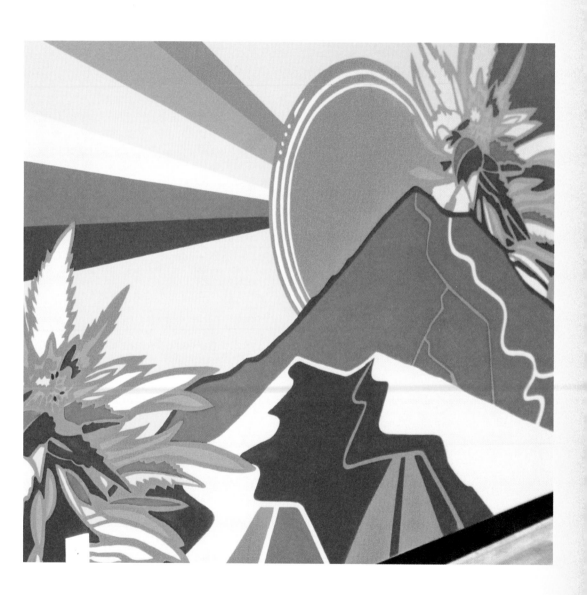

MOUNTAIN GIRL CANNABIS

THE FIRST LICENSED ADULT-USE CANNABIS STORE IN VERMONT ROOTED IN THE UTMOST LOCAL PRIDE.

When Ana and Josh MacDuff were granted the first retail license of Vermont's adult-use program, they took the honor and responsibility seriously. Recognizing how retail spaces were on the front lines of destigmatizing this plant, they took extra care when transforming a former auto parts store into a cozy, professional pot shop. They hung paintings of the surrounding mountains and natural views to soften the industrial space and sat glass jars with real flower on the counter for your aromatic perusal. You can bring your own mason jars in here for your flower purchase as well, just like filling a growler at your neighborhood pub. They'll even give you a discount!

The store's name is born in part from the founders' deep appreciation for the work and legacy of Carolyn Garcia, an advocate for sustainable cannabis cultivation and policy reform who is often referred to as "Mountain Girl," reflecting Vermont's nickname of the Green Mountain State, which the founders have called home for years. Love for their regional land shines through on the shop's shelves, too, where they're proud to carry flower from many of the state's most beloved farms, including Fierce Cultivation and Forbins Finest. There's also a solid array of blown glass pieces by local studio Haze Glass and satisfying edibles like the infused root beer-flavored hard candies from Tir Na Nog, a company founded by a pair of brothers and sixth generation Vermonters.

Whenever you visit Mountain Girl Cannabis, make sure to head into the nearby Giorgetti Park for all levels of hikes and start falling in love with the Green Mountain State yourself.

Open Daily

**174 West Street
Rutland, VT 05701**

mountaingirlcannabis.com

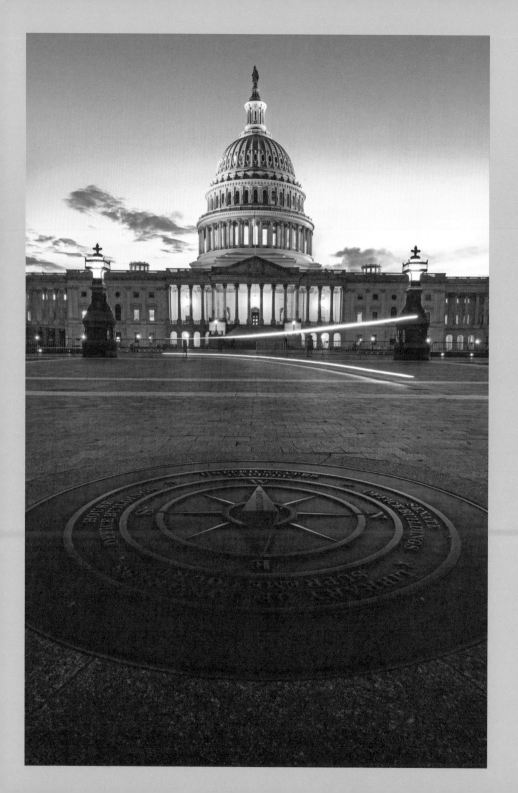

OTHER
LEGAL

As I mentioned in the introduction, this book doesn't include every US state that has legalized cannabis; rather it covers the states with the most developed and popular cannabis scenes. Naturally, this list will evolve over time. Alaska, for example, is a long-established market compared to New York, but are people traveling to Alaska exclusively for its cannabis?

Not quite yet. It takes a special combination of time, legislative support, and creative entrepreneurs to foster a dynamic community of cannabis businesses, and the following states, while legalized, are still working toward a more experiential scene.

STATES

ALASKA

LEGALIZED
Medical in 1998,
recreational in 2014

POSSESSION
Adults over the age of 21
can possess up to one
ounce of cannabis, seven
grams of concentrate,
or 5,600 milligrams of
edible THC.

HOME GROWS
Adults may grow up to six
mature plants at a time.

DELIVERY
Not legal

CONSUMPTION
Smoking is allowed on
private property or in
licensed consumption
lounges.

THE VIBE
From Seward to Palmer, and especially in Anchorage, dispensaries are established
and poppin'. In Juneau, the first consumption lounge, Cannabis Corner, has opened,
providing a vital public space for the community to connect and build. I'm looking
forward to seeing someone get weed-friendly nature experiences in motion.

CONNECTICUT

LEGALIZED
Medical in 2012,
recreational in 2021

POSSESSION
Adults over the age
of 21 can possess
1.5 ounce of cannabis,
7.5 grams of concentrate,
or 750 milligrams of
edible THC.

HOME GROWS
Adults may grow up to
three mature and three
immature plants at a time.

DELIVERY
Yes!

CONSUMPTION
Smoking is allowed on
private property.

THE VIBE
Dispensary sales are relatively new here at the time of writing, but Hartford is
already creeping up the list of interesting, cannabis-friendly cities in the making.
One thing the state has been ahead of the game on is automatically expunging
low-level, cannabis-related crimes. Major props to Governor Ned Lamont for
getting their "clean slate" law in motion right as adult-use sales kicked off.

DELAWARE

LEGALIZED
Medical in 2011, recreational in 2023

POSSESSION
Adults over the age of 21 can possess one ounce of flower, up to twelve grams of hash, or up to 750 milligrams of edibles.

HOME GROWS
Not allowed.

DELIVERY
Not legal (for now)

CONSUMPTION
Smoking is allowed on private property only.

THE VIBE
The cannabis scene here is yet to be determined as retail sales haven't quite kicked off yet. Visit the Marijuana Policy Project for the latest on legislative updates and rollout: mpp.org/states/delaware.

MARYLAND

LEGALIZED
Medical in 2013, recreational in 2022

POSSESSION
Adults over the age of 21 can possess up to 1.5 ounces of cannabis flower, twelve grams of concentrate, or a total amount of cannabis products that does not exceed 750 milligrams.

HOME GROWS
Adults may grow up to two plants.

DELIVERY
Yes

CONSUMPTION
Smoking is allowed on private property only and potentially at licensed consumption lounges (Ceylon House is a lounge that currently serves medical patients).

THE VIBE
Retail recreational sales haven't quite started yet, but the long established medical market bodes well for a cool and diverse scene to emerge. Visit the Maryland Cannabis Administration website for the latest: mmcc.maryland.gov.

OTHER LEGAL CITIES

MISSOURI

LEGALIZED

Medical in 2018, recreational in 2022

POSSESSION

Adults over the age of 21 can possess up to three ounces of flower or its equivalent in concentrates, vapes, or edibles form.

HOME GROWS

Adults may grow up to eighteen plants at a time. The catch is you have to register for a "consumer cultivator" card.

DELIVERY

Yes, medical only

CONSUMPTION

Smoking is allowed on private property only.

THE VIBE

Retail sales are just now getting underway, but the concentration of universities here implies a vibrant scene to come. Visit the Missouri Department of Health's website for the latest: cannabis.mo.gov.

RHODE ISLAND

LEGALIZED

Medical in 2006, recreational in 2022

POSSESSION

Adults over the age of 21 can possess up to an ounce of flower or its equivalent in concentrates, vapes, or edibles form.

HOME GROWS

Adults may grow up to six plants at a time.

DELIVERY

Not legal

CONSUMPTION

Smoking cannabis is now legal everywhere cigarettes are permitted. I'm jealous!

THE VIBE

For a small state, there's a broad spectrum of cannabis philosophies to be found in Rhode Island. While very strict jail time was still enforced for large possession charges well into the 2010s, the long-established medical scene belies that an open-minded community exists—open enough for The Healing Church in Rhode Island to operate a religious sect that treats cannabis as a holy part of their practice. I'm excited to watch this scene further develop.

VIRGINIA

LEGALIZED
Medical in 2020, recreational in 2021

POSSESSION
Adults over the age of 21 can possess one ounce of cannabis or the THC equivalent in other forms.

HOME GROWS
Adults may grow up to four plants at a time.

DELIVERY
Not legal

CONSUMPTION
Smoking is allowed on private property only.

THE VIBE
As of February 2023, the rollout of the recreational program is indefinitely on hold due to disagreements between state legislators. Visit the Virginia Cannabis Control website for the latest updates: cca.virginia.gov.

WASHINGTON, DC

LEGALIZED
Medical in 2011, recreational in 2015

POSSESSION
Adults over the age of 21 can possess up to two ounces of flower, five grams of concentrate, or sixteen ounces of edibles.

HOME GROWS
Adults may grow up to three mature plants and three seedlings at a time.

DELIVERY
Yes

CONSUMPTION
Smoking is allowed on private property only.

THE VIBE
The District of Columbia is a weird one. Although cannabis possession and consumption is legal, buying and selling it is not. This has resulted in a scene filled with "gifting shops" that get around the rules by selling items like a $40 T-shirt that happens to include a "free gift" in the form of an eighth of flower. Regardless, there is a scene of consumption-friendly spaces emerging, but it seems the Capital is not 100 percent on board with making sales officially legal just yet.

INDEX

ABOUT THE AUTHOR

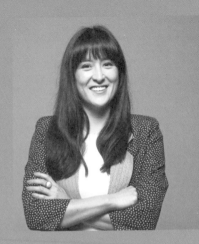

Lauren Yoshiko is a dedicated cannabis journalist from Portland, Oregon. When Oregon legalized adult-use cannabis in 2014, Lauren wrote some of the first articles about the industry. Technically, her career started a bit before then, during which she published strain reviews in Portland's Pulitzer Prize-winning alt-weekly, Willamette Week, under the pseudonym "Mary Romano" (Long story.) While she followed the evolution of cannabis business and culture for outlets like *Forbes*, *Broccoli Magazine*, Thrillist, Conde Nast, and *Rolling Stone*, she worked at dispensaries and a cannabis farm. She co-hosted Broccoli Magazine's podcast, Broccoli Talk, and continues to report on the evolving realm for various outlets and for Sticky Bits—her weekly newsletter for creative cannabis entrepreneurs.

PHOTO CREDITS

Cover image Wyllow; page 5 La Osa; 7 Leon Villagomez; 9 Kiskanu; 11 Nik Zvolensky; 13 Victor Pinho; 14 (top) Big Bad Wolf; 14 (bottom) Kenya Frank; 16 Posh Green Cannabis; 18 Nouera; 22 Amber Senter; 25 (top left and bottom) Damien Maloney; 25 (top right) Rose Los Angeles; 26 Diana Dalsasso; 29 Gorilla RX Wellness; 31 Highlites; 32 Josephine & Billie's; 35 Mister Green Life Store; 37 The Artist Tree; 38 Cannabis Supper Club; 41 Evan James; 43 (top) Chef Wendy Zeng; 43 (bottom) Bailey Robb; 44 Wyllow; 47 (top left and right) Madison Lawler; 47 (bottom) New Rituals; 49 Cornerstone Wellness; 51 Hicksville Pines Chalets & Motel; 55 Nayeli Gutierrez; 57 March and Ash; 61 Carefree Cannabis; 62 Olivia Ashton; 65 Green Muse; 67 Make and Mary; 68 Home Grown Apothecary; 71 Nomsternailz; 73 Somewhere; 74 Liz Vasquez; 76 Oregrown; 79 Tokyo Starfish's Bud and Breakfast; 81 Magic Number; 82 TokinTree House; 87 (top) Nichole Graf; 87 (bottom) Raven Grass; 89 (top) Chimacum Cannabis Company; 89 (bottom) Austin Brown; 90 Prism; 93 Heylo; 95 Dockside Dispensary; 96 CANNASWET; 99 Kimberley Bevington; 101 Canna West; 103 Mountain Views Tree House Joint; 104 Joint Rivers; 109 Juniper Cannabis; 111 Haskill Creek Farms; 116 Winona Grey; 119 Giving Tree; 121 The Clarendon Hotel and Spa; 123 Dino Jagger; 125 Sunday Goods; 127 Botanica; 130 Jacqueline Collins; 133 Shutterstock; 134 Wanda James; 137 Colorado Cannabis Tours; 138 Coryn Nelson Photography; 143 Dabsel Adams; 145 (top left and bottom) Dalwhinnie Farms; 145 (top right) Ahrling Photography; 148 Planet 13; 151 Tiffany Salerno; 153 The Lexi; 156 Carver Family Farms; 159 Rising Roots; 160 Wo Povi Cannabis; 163 Lava Leaf Organics; 165 Bighorn Weed Co.; 171 Dispensary 33; 172 Ivy Hall; 175 (top) Brianna Lotfy; 175 (bottom) Wake-N-Bakery; 177 Grasshopper Club; 178 West Town Bakery and OKAY Cannabis; 181 Herbal Notes; 183 Chitiva; 189 LIV Cannabis; 190 Falling Leaves Events; 193 Lucky Pistil Catering; 194 Jacob Lewkow; 196 Jessica Jackson; 199 Information Entropy; 200 Winewood Organics; 203 The Refinery; 209 Meowy Jane; 212 SeaWeed Co.; 219 (top) Sara Wallach; 219 (bottom) Farnsworth Fine Cannabis; 221 Rebelle; 222 Canna Provisions; 225 The Heritage Club; 227 Ciara Crocker; 228 Rooted In; 231 Sacrilicious; 233 (top) Botera; 233 (bottom) Chyanne Bessette; 234 Bud's Goods & Provisions; Summit Lounge; 239 Fine Fettle; 242 Live Love Lens Photography; 245 The Apothecarium; 247 Ebony Johnson; 250 Higher Standards; 253 Prince Franco; 254 Vic Styles; 257 Tricolla Farms; 258 (top) Black Owned Brooklyn; 258 (bottom) Happy Buds; 261 Higher Dining; 263 (top left) Marques Ruiz; 263 (top right) Daniela Villarreal; 263 (bottom) Pablo Isaak Perez; 264 The House of Cannabis; 267 Union Square Travel Agency; 269 Bend & Blaze Yoga; 270 Gotham/ Christopher Coe; 275 Daniel Schechner; 277 Magic Mann; 278 Mountain Girl Cannabis; 280 Shutterstock.

Published in 2024 by Hardie Grant Explore,
an imprint of Hardie Grant Publishing

Hardie Grant Explore (Melbourne)
Wurundjeri Country
Building 1, 658 Church Street
Richmond, Victoria 3121

Hardie Grant Explore (Sydney)
Gadigal Country
Level 7, 45 Jones Street
Ultimo, NSW 2007

www.hardiegrant.com/au/explore

Maps in this publication incorporate data from the
following sources: Made with Natural Earth. Free
vector and raster map data @naturalearthdata.com

A catalogue record for this
book is available from the
National Library of Australia

Hardie Grant acknowledges the Traditional Owners of
the Country on which we work, the Wurundjeri People
of the Kulin Nation and the Gadigal People of the Eora
Nation, and recognises their continuing connection to
the land, waters and culture. We pay our respects to
their Elders past and present.

Green Scenes
ISBN 9781741178883

10 9 8 7 6 5 4 3 2 1

Publisher
Megan Cuthbert
Editor
Lyric Dodson
Proofreader
Collin Vogt
Cartographer
Emily Maffei

Design
George Saad
Typesetting
Megan Ellis
Index
Max McMaster
Production coordinator
Simone Wall

Colour reproduction by Megan Ellis and
Splitting Image Colour Studio

Printed in China by 1010 Printing International Limited